THE EDUCATOR'S GUIDE TO STUDENTS WITH EPILEPSY

ABOUT THE AUTHOR

Robert J. Michael is the Chairperson of the Department of Educational Studies at the State University of New York, New Paltz, New York. He teaches undergraduate and graduate courses in the special education program at the college. Dr. Michael received his undergraduate degree from Farmington State College in Farmington, Maine, his Masters degree from the University of Southern California, a Certificate of Advanced Study from the State University of New York, and the Doctor of Philosophy degree from Fordham University.

He resides in Pine Bush, New York, with his wife Diann and three children, Rob, Holly, and Jenna.

THE EDUCATOR'S GUIDE TO STUDENTS WITH EPILEPSY

By

ROBERT J. MICHAEL
State University of New York
New Paltz, New York

CHARLES C THOMAS • PUBLISHER
Springfield • Illinois • U.S.A.

Published and Distributed Throughout the World by

CHARLES C THOMAS • PUBLISHER
2600 South First Street
Springfield, Illinois 62794-9265

ISBN 0-398-06537-3 (cloth)
ISBN 0-398-06538-1 (paper)

Library of Congress Catalog Card Number: 95-16962

With THOMAS BOOKS *careful attention is given to all details of manufacturing and design. It is the Publisher's desire to present books that are satisfactory as to their physical qualities and artistic possibilities and appropriate for their particular use.* THOMAS BOOKS *will be true to those laws of quality that assure a good name and good will.*

Printed in the United States of America
SC-R-3

Library of Congress Cataloging-in-Publication Data

Michael, Robert J.
The educator's guide to students with epilepsy / by Robert J. Michael.
p. cm.
Includes bibliographical references and index.
ISBN 0-398-06537 3 (cloth).—ISBN 0-398-06538-1 (paper)
1. Epileptic children—Education—United States. 2. Epilepsy.
I. Title.
LC4596.M53 1995
371.91′6—dc20

95-16962
CIP

To Diann,
Rob, Holly, and Jenna.

PREFACE

In the last two decades a major interest in education has been with students with disabilities. Litigation, legislation, and increased awareness have been hallmarks of the movement. However, there still remains a general lack of knowledge among educators concerning certain disorders that frequently can be found in children. This may be attributed to attitudes, misinformation, and lack of training.

One such disorder is epilepsy—one of the more common neurological conditions seen in today's classrooms. Although the Epilepsy Foundation of America (1987) states that about one in a hundred students have epilepsy, Freeman, Vining, and Pillas (1990) estimated that almost ten percent of the total population will experience a single seizure at some point in their life. Within the U.S. population of children aged 5 to 14 years old, 150,251 to 324,961 estimated new cases of epilepsy per year are projected (Hauser & Hesdorffer, 1990). Epilepsy is, indeed, an important developmental disorder among children.

Educators can make a commitment to provide the most appropriate and accepting educational program for the student with epilepsy. By recognizing that behavioral and academic problems may be associated with a child's particular disorder, programs can be established to meet the needs of the particular student.

There is a need to have educators become more aware of and knowledgeable about epilepsy. The purposes of this book are to:

(1) Present relevant knowledge about epilepsy for the educator;
(2) Create an awareness of and sensitivity to students with epilepsy;
(3) Focus attention on the role of education with students with epilepsy;
(4) Present the major educational issues associated with epilepsy;
(5) Define the educator's responsibility to students with epilepsy; and
(6) Present useful resources.

It is hoped that this book will help educators, parents, and other school personnel assist students who have epilepsy to become successful in school and in life.

The book is divided into eleven chapters. The first chapter presents an overview of epilepsy, emphasizing basic information and data about seizure disorders. The second chapter describes each type of seizure disorder, while the third chapter discusses the current challenges facing educators who work with students with special needs. The next section describes the essential components of major legislation that affect the lives of persons with epilepsy, while the fourth chapter discusses the role of the schools with students with epilepsy. Chapter 6 examines the student with epilepsy as a learner as well as focusing on epilepsy accompanying other disabilities. Chapter 7 presents specific strategies for increasing a student's self-esteem, as well as dealing with acceptance and understanding of this condition by students. Chapter 8 presents educators with an overview of medications used to treat students with epilepsy and the record keeping procedures that accompany it. Safety procedures, first-aid skills, and safe school environments highlight the following chapter, while Chapter 10 is concerned with the impact of epilepsy and the educator's roles of communicating and working with the family. The last chapter discusses the various forms of advocacy and the role of the educator.

Interspersed throughout the text are sections referred to as "FROM THE CLASSROOM" and "RESOURCES." In "FROM THE CLASSROOM" there are quotes, vignettes, and classroom examples about students with epilepsy. In "RESOURCES," useful materials, videos, organizations, and advocacy groups are presented for the benefit of educators and other school personnel who wish to create a better educational environment for the student with epilepsy.

Readers are cautioned not to make any medical changes based on the information in this book. Medical personnel must be consulted regarding the treatment of any person. There are also legislative mandates, changes in medical information, and technological advances that are being made continuously, and it is the educator's responsibility to keep aware of these changes.

The reader is also reminded that the intent and direction of this book is a reflection of this particular author's training and experiences. It is hoped that educators (in fact, all school personnel) will find this book useful as well as practical in meeting the needs of students with epilepsy.

I wish to acknowledge the help and support of a number of individuals.

I am especially grateful to former graduate students, Jean Herring, Ann Hazelnis, Christine Cook-Tierney, Paige Sedlak, and Cara Viggiano, for their extensive library and/or field work concerning students with epilepsy. Recognition is also given to Sandra Parks-Trusz for advice and feedback on the book. Particular appreciation is given to Lynn Van Eseltine Sarda for her constant encouragement and skilled guidance throughout the writing of this book. I also acknowledge the quotes, resources, and ideas shared by teachers, school nurses, school administrators, families, and colleagues from the Epilepsy Foundation of America.

R.J.M.

CONTENTS

THE EDUCATOR'S GUIDE TO STUDENTS WITH EPILEPSY

Chapter 1

OVERVIEW OF EPILEPSY

INTRODUCTION

DID YOU KNOW THAT . . .

- *There are over two million Americans with epilepsy?*
- *There are about one hundred and twenty-five thousand new cases of epilepsy that occur each year?*
- *Most individuals with epilepsy can be helped with medications?*
- *There are over twenty kinds of seizures associated with epilepsy?*
- *One of the most significant problems associated with epilepsy is people's attitudes?*
- *Everyone maintains a certain degree of susceptibility to seizures?*
- *There are over 300,000 students with epilepsy in schools in the United States?*

Epilepsy is a word derived from the Greek term *epilepsia* which means "to seize." It is a disorder of the brain with the major characteristic being recurrent seizures. The condition is a malfunctioning of the brain due to an electrical outburst within the cells. These recurrent discharges affect the normal operation of the nervous system. The result of this electrical "storm" within the brain is a seizure.

The seizure is a reaction of the body to the abnormal electrical outbursts within the brain. Not all seizures, however, are the result of epilepsy. For example, low blood sugar, infection, and fever can cause seizures but the person does not have epilepsy. When seizures recur, when they are unpredictable and without apparent medical cause, it may be epilepsy. Seizures that result in motor disturbances are labeled convulsions. However, seizures may involve disturbances in mental or physical areas of the body or both. Trained medical personnel will make the diagnosis and treatment plan with the family.

Although most occurrences of epilepsy are idiopathic (no known cause), there are instances when a direct cause can be attributed or hypothesized. Some known causes of epilepsy include lack of oxygen at birth, infectious diseases, poisons, strokes, head injuries, genetic factors, drug use, chromosomal abnormalities, and health problems during the pregnancy. In most cases, there is no direct reason why a person may have epilepsy.

Seizure threshold refers to the "susceptibility of a person to have seizures" (Epilepsy Foundation of America, 1991, p. 14). A low threshold indicates that a person would be more apt to experience a seizure. There are a number of factors which could affect a person's threshold. Heredity, photosensitivity (flashing lights), extreme fatigue, stress, hormonal changes and growth periods, and missed medication are significant factors. Others, which an educator should be familiar with, include head injury, fever, drug and alcohol use and illness. All people are unique individuals and not all are affected in the same way. How one handles these different factors varies from person to person. And only some seizures are influenced by these factors. Other seizures cannot be controlled by the person or the environment. Educators are in daily contact with students and are in an ideal situation for observing potential influences on seizures.

PREVALENCE

About two million people in the United States have epilepsy and about three-quarters of the cases start before age eighteen (Dreifuss, 1988). Hauser (1994) stated that about one hundred and fifty thousand children and adolescents in the United States will seek medical assistance each year for some type of seizure disorder. Freeman, Vining, and Pillas (1990) stated that almost ten percent of the total population will experience a single seizure at some point in their lives. However, they noted that 50 to 75 percent of those individuals having a seizure will not have another one. Persons who have isolated seizures will not be classified as having epilepsy, since the event is not repeated (Batshaw & Perret, 1986).

The Epilepsy Foundation of America (1987) estimated the prevalence of epilepsy to be about one percent of the total population. This factor varies a great deal in the literature due to the recognition that there is a reluctance to disclose because of stigma and prejudice associated with this disorder. Recognizing that there are numbers of individuals with epilepsy that have no official diagnosis or are now seizure-free and not seeing any medical personnel, Baroff (1991) puts the estimate of between 1 and 2 percent of individuals who ever experienced recurring seizures.

Students with epilepsy frequently are found in many of today's classrooms, schools, and agencies. In one study, 91 percent of the educational staff surveyed stated that they had medically fragile students in their classroom at some time. The educators who had students that were medically fragile reported that the most frequent health concern was seizures, as 64 percent of the educators stated that they had come into contact with students with this condition (Krier, 1993).

INCIDENCE

Cumulative incidence refers to the chance of an individual developing a particular disorder over a certain time period. Hauser and Hesdorffer (1990) noted that over one's lifetime, "the risk of developing epilepsy ranges from 1.4% to 3.3%" (p. 18). The authors noted that "on average, at least 1% of children can be expected to have an afebrile seizure by 14 years of age" (p. 31).

ONSET

Seizures can occur at any time and at any age. The highest rate of occurrence is for the group of individuals under 20 years old (Hauser & Hesdorffer, 1990). According to the Epilepsy Foundation of America (1981), 75 percent to 90 percent of individuals with epilepsy will experience their first seizure prior to age twenty. Ziegler (1982) noted the three most common time periods when epilepsy appears: 0–2 years of age, 5 to 7 years, and the early portion of puberty. Epilepsy can occur at any age, but it is most often known to appear in childhood (Jan, Ziegler, & Erba, 1983). However, the onset of some forms of epilepsy is related to the age of the child. Overall, the rate for children was highest in the less than two years of age group (Hauser & Hesdorffer, 1990), with the highest being in the first year of life (Hauser, 1994).

In the first five years of life, the majority are generalized seizures, but after this time it is partial seizures for about fifty percent of the new cases (Hauser, 1994).

ETIOLOGY

There is no definitive answer as to why brain cells fire abnormally in certain situations. Epileptologists often refer to two general areas of etiology: symptomatic and idiopathic (Baroff, 1991). Symptomatic refers to conditions associated with brain problems and disease, while idiopathic means that there is no known cause. About two-thirds of all cases of epilepsy are idiopathic (Hauser & Hesdorfer, 1990), and "in approximately half the cases of childhood-onset epilepsy with an identified cause for their epilepsy, the underlying condition is mental retardation or cerebral palsy (Hauser, 1994, p. s4).

Some individuals have an extreme sensitivity to flashing lights which may trigger seizures. This somewhat rare condition has been termed as "photosensitivity." Strobe lights, flickering computer monitors, flashbulbs from cameras, and video games have been named as possible triggers in some people. The Epilepsy Foundation of America has estimated that about three percent of all persons with epilepsy may have this sensitivity.

Some video game companies (i.e. Nintendo, Sega) have acknowledged that the flashing lights in the games may result in seizures in some people (Sullivan, 1994). The frequency of reporting seizures associated with video games may be underestimated (Graf, Glass, Knauss, & Chatrian, 1992). Additionally, flashing lights on fire alarms in buildings, a visual system created for warning persons with hearing impairments, have resulted in individuals experiencing seizures (Sullivan, 1994).

Some of the more known causes of epilepsy include: birth trauma, prematurity, anoxia, blood incompatibility, infections, genetics, brain infections, head injuries, poisons, metabolic disorders, and brain dysfunctions. With respect to age, seizures that begin before age two are usually associated with developmental disorders, injuries at birth, metabolic disorders, and/or infections. Seizures that begin when individuals are teenagers or in the early twenties are often related to head injuries and use of drugs or alcohol, if a cause is known. In fact, "an increasing number of seizures are attributable to illicit drug use, leading some neurologists to recommend drug screening in any adolescent or young adult with a first seizure" (Dodson, Leppik, & Pedley, 1991, p. 165). After this age, first seizures are associated with vascular problems and brain tumors. The list of possible causes could continue endlessly. Determining the possible cause is a medical endeavor and it is said that finding the exact cause is often not possible. Educationally, etiology of epilepsy has limited, if any, practical significance.

FROM THE CLASSROOM:

> **[An elementary school teacher states . . .] "I really don't fully understand everything that I should about epilepsy. All I know is that I treat her just like any other child. I really don't want her to stand out from the other children. She's just another child in the classroom."**

GENDER

The rates of epilepsy are higher in males than in females. This is possibly due to males acquiring more head injuries or because of the higher incidence of congenital anomalies (Hauser & Hesdorffer, 1990).

EPILEPSY AMONG MINORITIES

There is a greater frequency of epilepsy among black individuals than white (Hauser & Hesdorffer, 1990). However, other factors could enter into the data, "such as a potential increased risk of head injury and poorer perinatal care in lower socioeconomic status populations" (Hauser & Hesdorffer, 1990, p. 39).

Other populations of individuals need to be examined in future incidence and prevalence studies. This data could lead to other conclusions about the frequency of epilepsy in minority populations.

PERSONALITY

In past literature, an "epileptic personality" has been discussed. More recently, the notion that individuals with epilepsy may have particular personality or character traits has been cast aside. "Epilepsy presents the same range of personality and behavioral problems as is found in the general population, particularly in those with chronic illnesses" (Dreisbach, Ballard, Russo, & Schain, 1982, p. 114).

Particular forms of epilepsy, such as temporal lobe epilepsy, may lead a person to a certain personality type or set of characteristics. However, changes in personality by an individual with epilepsy could occur due to the behaviors of other persons directed to that individual (Dreisbach et al., 1982). Although the notion of a particular personality type has been discarded, there can, indeed, be an *effect* by epilepsy on a person's character.

SEIZURE COMPONENTS

The stages of a seizure are termed preictal, meaning the beginning, the seizure itself, and postictal, meaning the recovery.

Some individuals can sense the arrival of a seizure by the aura. This seizure signal could be sensed by an odd taste in the mouth, a peculiar smell, a specific vision, unique sounds, or a set of behaviors. It is extremely helpful if the educator knows (if possible) about the student's aura in order to assist and protect during the seizure activity. Peers also could be made aware of the impending seizure and, therefore, be available to assist their classmate.

An interesting sidelight to the information about auras has been the notion that dogs may be able to detect an aura before it occurs. According to Edney (1993), some dogs, prior to a person's seizure, displayed the following behaviors: anxiousness and/or restlessness, barking, whining, trying to get closer to the person, licking, and trying to get the person to lie down. According to Edney, dogs have also been known to react differently during the actual seizure. The author speculated that there may be particular odors given out by a person in an aura, which can be identified by some dogs.

EFFECT

Epilepsy as a disorder can be viewed as a mild inconvenience to a major disability. Along this continuum there are varying degrees of intrusion upon the student's life. There are also some factors that influence the effect of epilepsy on an individual:

Type: Seizures could be momentary stares or a full body convulsion with a loss of consciousness; the seizure activity could involve a small part of the brain or the total brain.

Frequency: Seizures could occur several hundred times a day or very rarely.

Duration: Seizures could be one second long or continuous, lasting many hours and requiring medical intervention.

Cause: Seizures could be caused from a variety of sources, such as diseases, poisons, metabolic imbalances, head injury, etc. Most seizures originate from unknown causes.

Behaviors: Seizures could trigger a finger or hand shaking, a stare, a full body convulsion, and automatisms such as lip smacking and picking at clothes to unconsciousness. There is no evidence of a greater amount of violence by persons with epilepsy compared to persons without epilepsy. There is a greater prevalence of epilepsy in prison populations, but it is similar to the prevalence rate within the lower socioeconomic population where prisoners often have lived (Treiman, 1986). Although a person with or without epilepsy could be violent, it is not a characteristic of the condition.

Verbalizations: During seizure activity individuals may keep verbal skills or lose them partially or totally. They may also express particular types of verbalizations. The responses for a person with consciousness include: being unable to speak, having slurred articulation, being unable to use language (aphasic), exhibiting stereotyped verbal responses (i.e., giving the same response to whatever question is posed), screaming or yelling at the start of a tonic-clonic seizure, producing sounds or screams during a partial seizure, emitting involuntary sounds, mumbling, or using profanity, and repeating other verbalizations stated by others (Lebrun, 1994).

Precipitants: Seizures may be brought on by a variety of stimulants, such as flickering lights, stress, certain sounds, etc. However, most seizures are unexpected and, in most cases, a particular trigger for a seizure cannot be defined.

Medication: Medications are used to control seizures. One drug or several different types of medications could be administered. One may get complete, partial, or no control over the seizure and the person may have severe, mild, or no side effects from the medication.

Other Disabilities: Students with seizures may have other disabilities, such as learning disabilities, autism, cerebral palsy or mental retardation. Some students with seizures may not have any other disabilities, and others may even be designated as gifted and talented. However, there is a higher incidence of epilepsy among individuals with other disabilities, such as autism, mental retardation, and cerebral palsy.

Stigma: Some students may be affected more by the stigma associated with epilepsy. In conjunction with stigma, various forms of discrimination are often experienced by those with epilepsy.

Kindling: There has been some discussion concerning the effect of uncontrolled seizures on the brain. If seizures keep occurring it is possible that a particular circuit or pathway for future seizures to occur is made. Driefuss (1988) refers to this intact connection within the brain as "kindling" (p. 7) and with this condition there may be an increased chance of the abnormal cell discharge to spread (Sands, 1982).

Impact: Students, peers, family, school personnel, etc. can influence the effect of epilepsy. Level of knowledge about epilepsy, acceptance, and attitude are important factors, among others, in determining the degree of impact of epilepsy. Epilepsy is a condition with the potential to impact on a person's quality of life. Variables concerning the quality of life for this population include: "health, family life, social, community and civic activities, personal development, and economics" (Hartshorn & Byers, 1992, p. 25). In a comparison study between children with epilepsy and children with asthma, it was determined that children with epilepsy had a more compromised quality of life in the psychological, social, and school domains (Austin, Smith, Risinger, & McNelis, 1994).

MYTHS AND STEREOTYPES

There are many myths and stereotypes concerning epilepsy. Individuals may encounter ideas, such as that persons with epilepsy:

- do not have a right to marry or to have children;
- cannot hold a job for any extended period of time;
- are mentally retarded;
- are possessed by evil spirits;
- are sick;
- are prone to commit crimes;
- need to be sheltered;
- are to be pitied;
- have hidden talents or hidden disabilities;
- may swallow their tongue during a seizure;
- have a condition that is contagious;
- possess an "epileptic personality" that is comprised of certain attitudes and behaviors related to the disorder.

Many of these myths originated in the past and have been carried through the years.

A LOOK TO THE PAST

Epilepsy is considered one of the oldest human disorders. In 2080 B.C. the Code of Hammurabi made reference to the marriages and the validity of court testimony by individuals with epilepsy (Bruya & Brolin, 1976). About four thousand years ago in the Near East, seizures were considered to be from demons or evil spirits. The idea of evil spirits in the body existed for many centuries and was embedded in many cultures. Individuals believed that making a hole in the skull would help cure a problem within the head. Skulls with varying size holes have been found throughout history.

During the time of Julius Caesar, epilepsy was known as "the falling disease." During this time a doctor named Galen suggested exercise, good diet, and the dissolving of phlegm (blockage within the brain) as a treatment for epilepsy. It was told that one of Galen's patients felt a cool breeze inside his body prior to a seizure. Galen named this feeling "aura" which means breeze in Greek (McGowen, 1989).

In ancient Greece, epilepsy was known as the "sacred disease" and if you had it the gods had touched you. When a person had epilepsy, it was considered divine. During the sixth century the Greeks moved away from the mythology associated with epilepsy and began studying disability rationally. Hippocrates examined disability through physiological factors, observing and recording objectively. He considered epilepsy to be a disease in the brain and not a magical condition. In fact, the first book about epilepsy, *On The Sacred Disease,* written by Hippocrates, noted that epilepsy was caused by a disturbance in the brain. "Through his efforts, retreats were established to habilitate persons with disabilities through rest, exercise, music, and other therapeutic activities" (Brimer, 1990, p. 4).

During the Middle Ages, religion was the framework for all activities. Disabilities were considered punishments for sins committed. A person with a disability was given mild exorcisms but at a later point during this time period harsher penalties, such as being starved, chained, or flogged, could be seen (Brimer, 1990). It was thought that these individuals needed the help of the saints. In fact, for a period of time the condition of epilepsy was referred to as St. John's disease (Geist, 1962).

At this time epilepsy was also referred to as "the demonic disease." Individuals with epilepsy were feared and often were driven away. It was often thought that epilepsy was contagious to the point that the breath of individuals with epilepsy was considered infectious (Scott, 1969). Persons with epilepsy were isolated and put into special hospitals that were more like prisons. Later, it was felt that seeing a person with epilepsy could trigger seizures in those who were looking (Scott, 1969).

Epilepsy was frequently related to mental retardation, and the people were treated in a similar manner (Smith & Luckasson, 1992). Thought to be caused by immoral behavior, the person with epilepsy was considered to be possessed by evil spirits. Many unusual treatments for epilepsy were created using religion, folklore, magic, and homemade concoctions.

In the 1700s many of the old ideas concerning epilepsy were discarded and many knowledge-based remedies were initiated. An attempt was made to get persons with epilepsy out of mental institutions, but many of the beliefs of the lay community persisted.

In most cases educational programs for students with disabilities consisted of care and shelter. Protection from the real world of cruelty, ridicule, pity, and rejection was the general practice. The origins of teaching students with disabilities were with European physicians.

One of the well-known physicians of this time was Jean Itard (1775–1838). Primarily known for his work with students who were deaf, the doctor began to work with a young boy about twelve years old who had been found in the woods of Aveyron, France. Apparently, the boy lived most of his life as a creature of the woods, acting and appearing in a feral state. Subsequently known as the Wild Boy of Aveyron, the child, named Victor, had no language or social skills. In addition, the Wild Boy had convulsions and spasms similar to epilepsy (Lane, 1976).

Itard was advised by his colleagues to abandon these efforts to educate this "hopeless idiot." He continued to work with the child, but after five years considered his project a failure, since the boy was still considered to have a disability. However, his work did improve Victor's behavior and he became more socialized, as well as having improved reading and writing abilities. Itard's work showed the use of systematic educational procedures with a child with a disability. Through the use of sound principles of learning, Itard illustrated that a person with a disability could learn.

One of Itard's students, Edouard Seguin, worked with children with mental retardation who, during these times, were regarded as being somewhat unteachable. The methodology, stressing sensory motor activities, used by Sequin to attempt to teach these children was based on Itard's work with Victor. These efforts became the framework for Maria Montessori's work in early childhood education and with children with mental retardation.

But the educational advances with students with epilepsy were still negligible. People often associated epilepsy with insanity. Despite the medical advances of the 1800s persons with severe epilepsy were placed in mental hospitals or locked into special wards of regular hospitals. It was during this time that the ideas that persons with epilepsy were dangerous and that the condition might be contagious were developed. Society was cruel and inhumane to this population of human beings. Survival was the key, with education playing a minor, if any, role.

Around the time of 1850, Sir Charles Locock, an English physician, found that bromide would control seizures in some individuals with epilepsy. McGowen (1989) noted that this was the only medicine for the treatment of epilepsy during this time. In the late 1800s, new discoveries were being made about epilepsy. During this time, Hughlings Jackson, a British neurologist, realized seizures were caused by a violent disturbance of the brain. He noted that certain seizures started with movements in one part of the body and then spread to other parts of the body in a systematic manner. This type of seizure was later called Jacksonian epilepsy.

Even in the early 1900s the literature, although thought to be accurate at that time, contained incorrect and inappropriate information about individuals with epilepsy. For example, Pressey and Pressey (1927) noted the critical need for institutional care for this population, since many "epileptics [*sic*] were at large" (p. 259). It was pointed out that one state colony in a particular area was quite inadequate and institutional care was not available. The authors noted that "in general the prognosis is rather poor. Treatment consists largely in eliminating the proteids from the patient's diet and in keeping the bowels open; this alone will often materially cut down the number of attacks" (p. 203).

Later, Scheidemann (1931) stated that learning for this population must take into consideration the intellectual abilities of the student, the severity of the disorder, and the vocational fields which may be open to those individuals with epilepsy. The author noted that "Epileptic children should be taught in special classes for their own sakes, as well as out of consideration for other children. The mortification experienced after a seizure, and the subsequent fear of another, disturbs a child greatly" (p. 484). In fact, educational programs for students with chronic conditions were created to meet the needs of the children with those specific disorders (Lynch, Lewis, & Murphy, 1992). The programs were located in special schools that isolated the students from their peers. During this time, the direction to take with this population can be best summarized by the following: "A quiet life, free from worry and excitement, with wholesome interests, and plenty of occupation, is the best treatment that can be provided" (Scheidemann, 1931, p. 484).

Prejudices, myths, and misunderstandings continued to affect individuals with epilepsy. In fact, McGowen (1989) noted that until the 1970s in many sections of the country it was a violation of law for a person with epilepsy to be married. Laws were enacted to prevent epilepsy from being passed to the children who would need to be institutionalized at taxpayers' expense. In a pamphlet distributed by the Epilepsy Foundation of America (1962), five states (Delaware, Nebraska, Utah, Virginia, and West Virginia) had laws related to marriage and people with epilepsy. According to the pamphlet, Delaware and West Virginia prohibited marriage by anyone with epilepsy, but the other states allowed marriage if sterilization or evidence of being cured was obtained. The laws were finally taken off the books, but the last one remained until 1982 (McGowen, 1989). In addition, immigration laws were changed. According to Sands and Minters (1977), "Before 1965, people with epilepsy were barred from the United States. In 1965, the Federal Immigration and Nationality Act was revised, and people with epilepsy were no longer excluded from the country" (p. 64).

Educationally, segregation of students with epilepsy persisted. In a booklet distributed from the U.S. Department of Health, Education, and Welfare (1961), it was stated that "You can see a child whose seizures are not controlled is out of place in a regular class" (p. 9). Several years later it was noted that educators were often reluctant to accept students with epilepsy into the schools, although it was recognized that this population belonged in the regular school system. In another booklet distributed by the U.S. Department of Health, Education, and Welfare (1964), it was stated that "In the past, many [persons with epilepsy] were kept at home or sent to special schools or institutions" (p. 17).

Throughout history there have been many famous people with epilepsy. Among the more well-known figures are Alexander the Great, Julius

Caesar, George Frederick Handel, Vincent Van Gogh, Napolean Bonaparte, Fyoder Dostoevski, and Pope Pius IX. However, their role in helping individuals with epilepsy become accepted was minimal, if any at all.

What do we see when we take a look to the past? Individuals with epilepsy were mistreated and neglected. It was a time for survival, with education and subsequent understanding and acceptance being the least of most people's concerns. As Tower (1960) stated, "most seizure patients are endorsed intellectually and could lead happy, useful lives if society would permit. But we are still haunted by the legacy of Roman and Medieval times that epilepsy is to many a socially unacceptable disease" (p. 9).

Chapter 2

TYPES OF SEIZURES

There are many kinds of seizures and they have varying effects. Epilepsy is a disorder that is comprised of over twenty types of seizures and, according to Bergen (1991), it is quite possible for children to experience more than one type of seizure, especially if brain injuries are involved.

The type of seizure depends on where it starts and the spread of the electrical discharge. In the past, seizures were classified as being either grand mal or petit mal. As the French word for big is grand, for small is petit, and bad is mal, we had a system referring to big and small seizures that were bad. This outdated terminology and classification system, possibly still used by some individuals, is not the current and accepted method of classifying seizures.

Seizures are divided into two main categories termed (1) generalized seizures and (2) partial seizures. The International Classification system breaks these categories into subgroups with the resulting benefits of facilitating communication, assisting with prescribing medications, and helping with the exchange of information about seizures (Dreifuss, 1988). Generalized seizures include absence seizures, myoclonic seizures, atonic or drop attacks, and tonic-clonic seizures. Partial seizures are divided into simple partial seizures and complex partial seizures. Generalized seizures have their origins within the brain and go through both sides of it. They involve an electrical outburst within most of the brain and usually involve some degree of loss of consciousness. Partial seizures, on the other hand, involve only a part of the brain. Figure 1 illustrates this classification of seizures.

ABSENCE SEIZURES

Formerly called petit mal seizures, absence seizures are the most common type of generalized seizures, as well as being a common seizure disorder of childhood (Murphy & Dehkharghani, 1994). They are

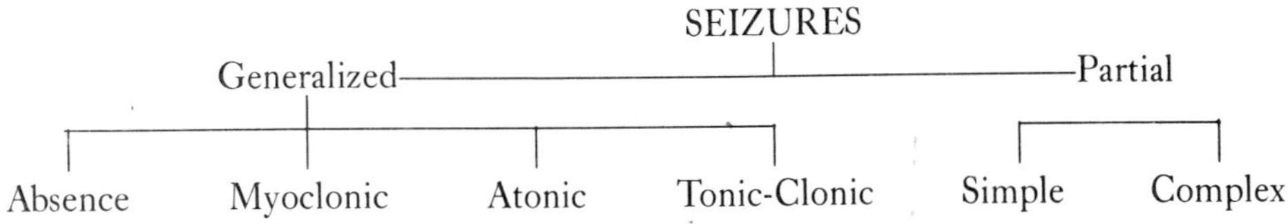

Figure 1. Classification of Seizures

characterized by short, brief interruptions in consciousness, usually lasting from 5 to 15 seconds with the person feeling normal after the seizure (Porter, 1993). An absence seizure may be seen as a stare, small movements of the eye, or fluttering of the eyelids. What a teacher might see varies, but in many cases the student blinks the eyes or drops the head slightly. The person might drop anything held in the hand. There may be some small involuntary movements or jerking motions. The student could be just staring blankly or having a glassy-eyed look. There is not any awareness during this time and generally there is no recall of events which occurred. Young adults with absence seizures have reported that one of the major impacts of the condition on their lives was difficulties in school achievement (Olson & Campenhausen, 1993). The student misses what is going on in the classroom and the teacher might think the student is daydreaming or just not paying attention. Michael (1992) stated, "Frequently, she would stare vacantly at the teacher, appearing not to understand what was occurring in the room. These expressionless, vacuous gazes became a serious concern for everyone involved with the child. The teacher noted that these short staring episodes were occurring more frequently, and the child often failed to acquire important information" (p. 211).

An absence seizure could last up to ten seconds and it is feasible to have one after another. Absence seizures begin in early childhood and may disappear as the person gets older. Generally, absence epilepsy begins between the ages of four and eight years of age (Murphy & Dehkharghani, 1994). There is evidence of a genetic predisposition to this condition, although it is not fully understood (Porter, 1993).

FROM THE CLASSROOM:

[A teacher notes . . .] "It's the subtle seizures that are a problem. They aren't obvious and you don't easily see them as seizures. It looks like the kids are not paying attention or that they

are a behavior problem. I wonder if these seizures are really noticed?

"I wondered about her paying attention in class. She seemed like she was in her own little world. The medical evaluation told us that she was having absence seizures—possibly hundreds on any given day."

MYOCLONIC SEIZURES

Myoclonic seizures are characterized by quick, sudden, muscular movements. These fast jerks can range from mild to severe and have different forms. For example, the student may throw a hand out or be totally thrown to the ground. These types of seizures "are like being jolted by an electric shock" (Freeman et al., 1990, p. 63). Myoclonic seizures are "very brief, sudden, shock-like muscular contractions that may occur alone or in clusters" (Murphy & Dehkharghani, 1994, p. s9).

ATONIC SEIZURES

Atonic seizures, also called drop attacks, are characterized by a quick loss of muscle tone. The muscles in the arms, legs, or body go limp. The student suddenly drops, loses consciousness, and falls to the ground. Recovery occurs generally after ten seconds to a minute (Epilepsy Foundation of America, 1991). This type of seizure can easily cause facial and head injuries. Protective helmets are often worn for safety.

FROM THE CLASSROOM:

[A teacher states . . .] "He just goes totally limp and drops to the floor. He is such a big kid that we have to be careful that he doesn't come down on somebody else."

TONIC-CLONIC SEIZURES

Formerly referred to as grand mal seizures, tonic-clonic seizures are characterized by convulsions and a loss of consciousness. They are the type most people think of when seizures are discussed. Tonic-clonic are the most common type of seizure in children.

What is usually seen is that the person loses consciousness and falls to the ground. The tonic phase is when the muscles of the body become stiff and very rigid. After this part, a clonic phase begins, characterized by the arms and legs jerking and moving very rapidly. If a screaming sound is heard, do not assume the person is in pain. Air rushing past the vocal cords when the muscles have contracted creates this sound. One might see the person exhibit a number of other behaviors during the seizure, such as teeth grinding, irregular breathing, saliva flow from the mouth, and a loss of bladder and/or bowel control. After the tonic-clonic seizure the person is generally very tired and could be quite disoriented or confused. It is not unusual for the person to experience a headache and need rest.

Michael (1992) described an incident for the benefit of educators:

> Susan began to feel irritable and queasy. Her lips began to turn a purplish tone and she felt quite lightheaded. Her facial skin coloring lost its natural glow and became exceptionally pallid. Susan fell to the floor and lost consciousness. Her total body began to shake, twist, and writhe, and saliva began to drip slowly from the corner of her mouth. Her eyelids quivered, and it appeared that her eyes were rolled back. Several minutes later, she stopped convulsing and awoke, feeling quite tired and weary. (p. 211)

SIMPLE PARTIAL SEIZURES

Simple partial seizures, sometimes referred to as focal or focal motor seizures, involve the moving or jerking of a particular part of the body. Depending on what part of the brain is involved with the seizure, that certain body part (i.e. face, hand, or leg) will be affected. It may also affect the senses, such as tingling or other abnormal feeling in a part of the body. Again, the jerking or feeling will depend on what part of the brain is experiencing the electrical discharge.

If the part of the brain that is affected is related to the visual sense, abnormal visual experiences occur, such as seeing things which are nonexistent. Other senses may also be affected. These sensory seizures result in a distorted environment. For example, the person may see various shapes and colors, smell unusual odors, or feel odd physical sensations. It is possible for the person to hear sounds which did not occur or experience fear, nausea, joy, or anger for no apparent reason.

During a simple partial seizure the person is conscious and aware throughout the experience. However, there is a possibility that it could spread to a convulsive seizure.

Freeman, Vining, and Pillas (1990) noted that partial seizures may spread slowly through the motor area. For example, a jerking finger turns to jerking of all the fingers, and then to the wrist and hand. At a later point, it could move to the arm and face. This type of seizure has been termed a "Jacksonian seizure" in the past, as Hughlings Jackson first observed the motor progression of the seizure.

Simple partial seizures have also been described with autonomic symptoms and with psychic symptoms (Freeman et al., 1990). A seizure can begin in a part of the brain that is concerned with involuntary functions such as the heartbeat. The authors describe an example of a simple partial seizure with autonomic symptoms when stating that "it may start with the face becoming pale and flush. The heart may begin to beat rapidly; there may be abdominal cramps and discomfort or a fullness in the chest or throat" (p. 76).

Simple partial seizures with psychic symptoms originate in the part of the brain dealing with emotions, feelings, and/or prior experiences. Dreifuss (1988) noted that if the temporal lobe portion of the brain is affected, feelings of unreality, fear, or anger, as well as disturbances in memory can occur. Freeman, Vining, and Pillas (1990) stated that the child may have a very frightened look, voices may be heard, sensations of déjà vu or jamais vu (never seen), as when something very familiar appears to be unknown.

COMPLEX PARTIAL SEIZURES

Complex partial seizures, sometimes referred to as temporal lobe seizures or psychomotor seizures in the past, are similar to simple partial seizures except that consciousness is disrupted or lost.

The seizure may begin with the person entering a dream-like state or having a blank stare. The person may exhibit some type of "automatic" type behaviors, such as mumbling, pulling or picking at one's clothes, lip smacking, chewing, removing one's clothes, walking around aimlessly, talking in a nonsense manner or performing simple random, purposeless activity. The individual may seem dazed and the activities of the seizure are not remembered. These seizures frequently are not recognized by educators and others (Santilli, Dodson, & Walton, 1991), and they are often misinterpreted as signs of substance abuse (Potolicchio, 1992). The seizure may last one to five minutes and the person could often appear to be confused at the end of the seizure.

In examining the behaviors involved with complex partial seizures with infants, Duchowny (1987) concluded that an elevated and extended arm, head turned toward the arm, lower extremities being flexed or extended, jerking eye or mouth movements, and facial automatisms "consisting of grimacing, lip smacking, chewing, and eye flutters" (p.911) could be seen. And, in order to classify these seizures as complex, a loss of awareness or consciousness was observed.

FROM THE CLASSROOM:

> **[A young adult states . . .] "I have complex partial seizures but often people don't notice them. In school I stayed in my seat and in my classroom. Everyone knew about them but really didn't pay much attention to them after awhile. I didn't want people to see them anyway. I didn't want to make a big deal out of it. I guess I must have missed some things in school, but I really wasn't a good student anyway. I'm not even sure if all the teachers even recognized all my seizures; maybe some of them didn't even know."**
>
> **[A teacher states . . .] "The student would have at least two or three per day. It didn't matter where or what she was doing—she would just drop everything and look totally lost."**

STATUS EPILEPTICUS

Status epilepticus is not a type of seizure disorder but is recognized as a particular condition. It is defined as a special circumstance when seizures follow each other without allowing the person to regain consciousness. Individuals in this condition experience seizure activity for at least thirty minutes (Murphy & Dehkarghani, 1994). Status epilepticus can often be a person's first seizure and it can occur at any age. However, this condition is more common with children and in elderly individuals. Status epilepticus occurs in about sixty thousand people annually. It is possible to have this condition with any type of seizure disorder, but the most common is tonic-clonic (Leppik, 1990).

If the status epilepticus seizures are tonic-clonic, the condition endangers the person's life (Driefus, 1988; Freeman et al., 1990) and is considered a medical emergency. Leppik (1990) stated the need for emergency medical care in order to prevent damage to the brain and/or possible death.

A nonconvulsive status is when a person has extensive staring spells or times of confusion lasting thirty minutes or longer (Freeman et al., 1990). Although the nonconvulsive condition is not life threatening, it has many implications for educators, as will be discussed later.

Leppik (1990) noted that numbers of persons with status epilepticus were not complying with their drug treatments. The importance of maintaining medical treatment for those with epilepsy was stressed.

RESOURCE:

Schachter, Steven G. *The Brainstorms Companion*

Epilepsy in our View. New York: Raven Press, 1995.

This small book contains descriptions of seizures in the words of family members, friends, and acquaintances.

EPILEPSY SYNDROMES

Syndromes are defined as a set of related characteristics associated with a particular condition. Symptoms or behaviors are grouped together with the seizure condition which create specific syndromes associated with epilepsy. Some syndromes can be quite benign while others can be quite severe and life threatening.

Examples of epilepsy syndromes include Lennox-Gastaut syndrome, Rolandic epilepsy, and infantile spasms. Lennox-Gastaut syndrome has mental retardation as a characteristic as well as cognitive deterioration (Dam, 1990). The age to acquire this condition is usually one to eight years old (Hauser & Hesdorffer, 1990). With having frequent and various types of seizures, along with mental retardation, the prognosis with this condition is considered poor (Hauser & Hersdorffer, 1990). Rolandic epilepsy is characterized by partial motor seizures, often happening in the night (Driefuss, 1988), while infantile spasms syndrome is a severe early childhood disability, classified within two different forms. In the idiopathic form "the seizures are characterized by sudden myoclonic jerks with flexing of the neck and body and stiffening of the limbs"

(Driefuss, 1988, p. 7). They are often seen as groups of jolting movements. In the symptomatic type, the outlook is not as good. With mental development affected, the long-term prognosis is poor (Dam, 1990).

With the various syndromes, "the underlying etiology is a determining factor for future intellectual development" (Dam, 1990, p. s28).*

FEBRILE SEIZURES

Febrile seizures are a type of seizure condition which is not epilepsy. This particular disorder is characterized by convulsions brought on by a rapid rise in body temperature. It is not epilepsy, as epilepsy has recurrent seizures with no precipitating factor such as fever. However, the seizure may look similar to a tonic-clonic seizure in that the child loses consciousness and experiences convulsions. Febrile seizures are separate from epilepsy but are related (Hopkins, 1981). Michael (1992) presented an example of this condition when stating:

> Awakening one morning, Harry, who is 3 years old, was quite irritable and lethargic. He complained that his ears ached and his head hurt. Later that morning, the day-care person found Harry unconscious on the floor, jerking and flailing his arms and legs. The thrashing, contorting movements lasted several minutes. When the convulsion had stopped, Harry was quite tired and needed rest. Harry was found to have to have two ear infections and a high fever. (p. 211)

Fishman (1979) stated that "simple or benign febrile seizures are characterized by lasting less than 15 minutes, by not having focal features, and by not occurring in a series which has a total duration greater than 30 minutes. Complex febrile seizures are those which are long in duration, focal, and occur in series" (p. 178).

Driefuss (1988) noted that febrile seizures are quite common, with 3 percent to 5 percent of the population being affected. Freeman, Vining, and Pillas (1990) stated that while febrile seizures are not usually seen in the child's first months, the number of children with the seizures is highest at about eighteen months and the seizures are usually outgrown by five years of age. Gorman and Snead (1979) stated that 40 percent of febrile seizures last less than five minutes while 75 percent of this type of seizure lasts less than 20 minutes. Genetic factors play a role in one's

*Additional information about epilepsy syndromes can be found in resources, such as Wyllie (1993), *The treatment of epilepsy: Principles and practice* (Philadelphia: Lea & Febiger), and Devinsky, O. (1994), *A guide to understanding and living with epilepsy* (Philadelphia: F.A. Davis).

susceptibility to febrile seizures as it is passed on through a dominant gene (Hopkins 1981).

The risk for developing epilepsy for all children (including those with neurologic complications) who had febrile seizures was about six percent (Annegers, Hauser, Elveback, & Kurland, 1979). The risk factors for subsequent development of epilepsy in a child who has had a single febrile seizure are:

- If the first febrile seizure is prolonged (more than fifteen minutes), if the seizure was one-sided or focal, or if there were two or more seizures during that episode;
- If there is a family history of epilepsy;
- If the child has a neurological disorder, such as cerebral palsy, or if his [*sic*] development had been delayed before the seizure. (Freeman, Vining, & Pillas, 1990, p.42)

According to the Consensus Statement (1980) made by a panel of experts, children with febrile seizures have a 30 percent to 40 percent risk of having other febrile seizures. In addition, they found only a slight increase in obtaining epilepsy. The panel also concluded that they found no evidence of impairment because of the seizures. More recently, Dodson, Leppik, and Pedley (1991) concurred when they stated that febrile seizures are not associated with intellectual or neurological impairments. The future for children with febrile seizures is deemed to be excellent (Cavazzuti, Ferrari, & Lalla, 1984; Murphy & Dehkharghani, 1994).

While some authors have stated that intelligence and learning are not affected by febrile seizures, Wallace (1984) found a higher incidence of learning and behavior problems by children with this condition. Smith and Wallace (1982) found that after a first febrile seizure, subsequent seizures were probably more harmful to overall intellectual development than the use of medication over time (phenobarbitone or sodium valproate). If there is a good chance of further seizures, the findings support the use of medication. If the child has a lowered chance of more seizures, the authors felt that medication should be avoided in light of the effects on intellectual development.

In another investigation, Wallace and Cull (1979) stated that in particular cases, repeated febrile seizures affected cognitive abilities. The results of the study indicated that boys had no damage but girls did, particularly if the seizures were unilateral. Damage, as measured by scores on the Bender Visual Motor Gestalt Tests, was evident with girls who had prolonged or repeated unilateral seizures. The authors stressed the use of anticonvulsant medications to prevent repeated and prolonged seizures.

However, most children with febrile seizures need no anticonvulsant medication. When a medication is prescribed, phenobarbital is the most commonly used medication for febrile seizures, as this drug has been shown to decrease the frequency of febrile seizures (Camfield, Camfield, Shapiro, & Cummings, 1980). Yet, 40 percent of children using phenobarbital display side effects such as hyperactivity, irritability, sleep disturbances, and interference with cognitive function (Consensus Statement, 1980).

The child with febrile seizures must be examined by a physician to rule out other conditions, such as meningitis. Uncomplicated febrile seizures usually do not require treatment, but recurring febrile seizures may necessitate drug therapy, such as the use of phenobarbital (Gorman & Snead, 1979). First-aid procedures, as practiced for tonic-clonic seizures, are used. Most often, the convulsions of febrile seizures stop in a few minutes and the child is not harmed. Early childhood educators must be aware of febrile seizures and knowledgeable about first-aid procedures.

NONEPILEPTIC SEIZURES

A nonepileptic seizure is an event that is similar to an epileptic seizure, but it is not created from abnormal neuron discharges that typically occur in epileptic seizures (Metrick et al., 1991). The behaviors associated with this condition have been called, in the past, hysterical seizures, pseudoepileptic seizures, etc. Although many of these names suggest a psychological base to these behaviors, they do not all originate from a psychological domain and can include a medical origin (Walker & Rowan, 1993). Panic, hyperventilation, migraines, and breath-holding spells are also, at times, mistaken for epileptic seizures (Dodson, Leppik, & Pedley, 1991). These goal-directed behaviors are not a part of seizure activity (Murphy & Dehkharghani, 1994). Other types of nonepileptic activity include night terrors and movement disorders (Murphy & Dehkharghani, 1994).

Some of the same characteristics of epileptic seizures can be seen with nonepileptic seizures. The consequences of such seizures are the same, with many of the same effects as epileptic seizures. Complicating the matter is the fact that an individual can experience both epileptic and nonepileptic seizures.

The basis of many treatment approaches uses the neurologist, psychologist/psychiatrist and the person with the condition as a team to establish care and treatment plans. However, these seizures have a number of causes and a number of types of treatment plans (Walker & Rowan, 1993).

FROM THE CLASSROOM:

> [A teacher states . . .] **"We thought for sure that he was having some kind of seizure. He would put his head down on the desk and be out of it for several minutes. This could happen quite often during the day or just occasionally. After the child was tested by a neurologist we found out that it wasn't epilepsy and it was narcolepsy (a sleeping disorder). Appropriate medication was prescribed for the child."**

SUMMARY

It is important to remember that students with seizures can exhibit a variety of behaviors. The appearance of the seizures differ, and there are a number of different types of the condition with which educators should be familiar. Some students lose consciousness; others don't. Some may get a warning that the seizure is coming and others may only have seizures at night or in the early morning. The major point is that seizures are different just like students are different. Seizures and their effects are not all the same.

RESOURCE:

Epilepsy Foundation Of America
4351 Garden City Drive
Landover, MD 20785

EFA Toll-Free Information Service
(800) EFA-1000

EFA National Library
(800) EFA-4050

The foundation provides information on research, resources, and services to persons and families with epilepsy.

Chapter 3

CURRENT CHALLENGES

Although there is a great deal of information about schools and education, current issues often affect many of our daily practices with students. The following section begins by presenting areas that are deemed critical for educators who want to establish appropriate programs for students with epilepsy. An understanding of these current challenges will put the education of this population of students into proper perspective. The following sections will deal with the philosophy of normalization, an understanding of handicapism, a definition of the least restrictive environment, the various views on inclusion, a brief explanation of the zero reject principle, a discussion of attitudes as they pertain to individuals with epilepsy, and a call for all educators to keep aware of the advances being made in the medical arena for the treatment of epilepsy.

NORMALIZATION

An important principle for educators who are working with students with epilepsy is normalization, a term developed by Wolfensberger (1972). Normalization is usually defined as a way of living and learning that is as close to normal as possible. Persons with a disability should be integrated into all aspects of life. Their lives should be as much like persons that are nondisabled.

The normalization movement has resulted in a number of changes in the way individuals with disabilities have been treated. For example, normalization has had educators move away from labeling of students. Individuals are more sensitive to the effects of referring to a person as mentally retarded, learning disabled, or epileptic. The civil rights of individuals with disabilities have also grown from this movement, as well as the development of a sensitivity to the stereotypes of disabilities. Deinstitutionalization and the moving of individuals with severe disabilities closer to living in their own neighborhoods, such as in group homes, have been recent trends and a result of normalization. Mainstreaming is the integration of students with disabilities into regular classrooms and away from self-contained, isolated environments, while the Regular Education Initiative (REI) is calling for regular classroom teachers to assume responsibility for the education of students with disabilities. Both mainstreaming and the REI call for changes that are aimed at making the lives of students with disabilities much more in line with the principles of normalization.

Students with epilepsy are, indeed, participating in the normalization movement. Unless another condition is present and necessitates additional educational changes, schooling for this population of students should be quite similar to that of other individuals. Normalization is aimed at enhancing the lives of persons with disabilities and is an important consideration when dealing with students with epilepsy.

Normalization also means that the person has the "dignity of risk" (Perske, 1972). Many students with disabilities, including those with epilepsy, are overprotected and not allowed the dignity of risks. Challenges of risk are necessary for human growth and development. The typical risks of living are a necessary part of life and students with epilepsy should be allowed to take chances for success or failure like other students.

The normalization movement provides opportunities for all students to be accepted in our nation's classrooms. It is time to stop rejecting students who are different. As Baroff (1991) aptly stated, "Xenophobia is not just an ethnic response to the stranger, it is also our individual one to persons who have characteristics we would not wish for ourselves, and about whom our lack of contact ensures the perpetuation of cultural stereotypes, fears, and propensities for avoidance" (p. 241).

FROM THE CLASSROOM:

[A teacher states . . .] "The emphasis must be on the normalcy of children with seizure disorders."

HANDICAPISM

Joining the many other "isms" (racism, ageism, sexism, etc.) is the word handicapism, a term originating from the disability activists' movement. Bogden and Biklen (1977) defined handicapism as "a set of assumptions and practices that promote the differential and unequal treatment of people because of apparent or assumed physical, mental, or behavioral differences" (p. 14). Similar in idea to racism and sexism, it can be viewed in terms of stereotyping, discrimination, prejudice, and devalued roles in society.

Wolfensberger (1985) offered a listing of groups of people who are devalued due to particular deviancy roles. The analysis showed that individuals with epilepsy would be treated poorly and are perceived in a very negative fashion. The common deviancy roles, according to Wolfensberger (1985), for persons with epilepsy included pity, charity, sickness, and dread. When individuals are perceived negatively, the treatment received from others is different and is often unequal.

FROM THE CLASSROOM:

(A teacher states . . .) "Safety and protection of the child are important issues, but don't lose sight of the child's need to be considered 'part of the group' and not singled out or coddled."

RESOURCE:

THE DISABILITY RAG
P.O. Box 145
Louisville, KY 40201

THE DISABILITY RAG is a publication that deals with disabilities as a civil rights issue. It attacks stereotypes, labeling, and misconceptions about persons with disabilities. The ***RAG*** is available in regular type, large print, or cassette.

LEAST RESTRICTIVE ENVIRONMENT

The Individuals With Disabilities Education Act (IDEA) defined least restrictive environment (LRE) as "that to the maximum extent appropriate, handicapped children . . . are educated with children who are not handicapped, and . . . removal from the regular educational environment occurs only when the nature or severity of the handicap is such that education in regular classes with the use of supplementary aids and services cannot be achieved satisfactorily" (Section 34 CFR 300.550).

Based on the particular needs of the student, a full continuum of program placement options must be made available. The options can range from the regular class to residential placement. The multidisciplinary placement team must examine the needs of each particular student, but an emphasis on using the regular classroom should be made. Recently, the courts have started to demand that schools implement the least restrictive environment with students with disabilities. "If school districts do not take the initiative to restructure their educational programs so that the LRE mandate can be implemented fully, they may be forced to do so under court orders" (Osborn & Dimattia, 1994, p. 13).

Although there have been many interpretations of the "least restrictive environment," students with disabilities must be educated "to the maximum extent appropriate" with students who do not have disabilities. Through such integration, students with epilepsy are not alienated and they have the opportunity to learn to deal and cope with other students. Everyone learns about epilepsy, and stigma and discrimination are, hopefully, reduced. The students learn from and about each other.

> **[A father of a student with epilepsy states . . .] "There is no reason why my child should be separated. He should be with the other children. They are his friends. Other kids need to know about disabilities. This is a good chance to learn about them and to learn about my son."**

INCLUSION

Inclusion is defined as students with disabilities being educated full time in the regular classroom. Salend (1994) stated that, "Inclusionary schools welcome, acknowledge, and affirm all learners by educating them together in high quality, age-appropriate, regular education classrooms in their communities" (p. 49). The students learn at their own rate and, as advocates of the movement state, lose the stigma of being "special." However, the inclusion movement can and does mean different things to different people, ranging from being nothing new to a total reorganization of schools (Fuchs & Fuchs, 1994).

The goal is to abolish special education as it presently operates and to promote students' social skills, as well as to create a change in attitudes of educators and students without disabilities (Fuchs & Fuchs, 1994). The current system of pulling students out of the classroom to receive special education services gives a piecemeal approach to programming (Hardman, Drew, Egan, & Wolf, 1993). With inclusion, special supports for students in the regular classroom would be maintained. "It [inclusion] involves bringing the support services to the child (rather than moving the child to the services) and requires only that the child will benefit from being in the class (rather than having to keep up with the other students)" (Rogers, 1993, p. 1).

> **[A mother of a student with epilepsy states . . .] "I hope the other children learn to be tolerant. I'm not sure if he'll be accepted, but I want to give it a try."**

ZERO REJECT PRINCIPLE

In the past, individuals with disabilities have been denied appropriate education and related services in the schools. More recently, appropriate educational placements and services have become a reality. Legislation and litigation have established the "zero reject" principle by stating that no child can be denied an education based on the degree or severity of the disability. Procedural rights and protections are given to students with disabilities and their parents/guardians. All students are entitled to the right to an appropriate education.

ATTITUDES

Attitudes toward individuals with disabilities have often been influenced by misinformation and/or lack of information. Our culture historically has segregated individuals who are viewed as different. Whether it has been through special programs or special classrooms or schools, systems have been created in order to segregate individuals with disabilities.

Language is a powerful tool that influences attitudes toward students with disabilities. Particular terms are considered outdated and offensive to use when communicating with and about persons with disabilities. For example, saying "the handicapped," "the disabled," "the mentally retarded," and "the epileptic" is considered condescending and groups students into a category. This type of language can create overgeneralizations which lead to stereotypes. Having a "fit" is particularly outdated when referring to a seizure.

Various images are developed by the labels put on people. Mentally retarded, epileptic, learning disabled are examples of labels that develop ideas of what a person is or is not. There is a need to have educators recognize the abilities of students, seeing past any labels that might influence attitudes. It is our responsibility to gain information about our students, to recognize any misinformation, and to correct it.

FROM THE CLASSROOM:

> **[A school nurse states . . .] "If we can get them [school personnel] to stop calling them fits, we'll have made some progress. It's really in poor taste, but most people don't really know."**

There are, indeed, other words that view students in terms of their disability. Crippled, disturbed, deaf and dumb, etc. are further examples of offensive terminology. It stigmatizes, dehumanizes and implies inferiority. In fact, the word "handicap" has often been thought to come from a time when individuals with disabilities were begging in the streets with a "cap in hand." "Disabled people resent words that suggest they are sick, pitiful, childlike, dependent, or objects of admiration . . . " (Shapiro, 1993, pp. 32–33).

Current practices in terminology concerning disabilities use phrases such as students with disabilities, children who are hearing impaired, and people with mental retardation. The person is named first and is then connected to the disability with a preposition (i.e., students with disabilities). As the Disability Advisory Council of Australia (1992) noted, "Prepositions, on the other hand, imply both 'a relationship to' and 'a separation from'. At this historical juncture the awkwardness in phrasing that often results may be all to the good, for it makes the user and the hearer stop and think about what is meant, as in the terms 'people of color' and 'persons with a disability' " (p. 58).

A student with epilepsy needs to be viewed as a person, not as a type of seizure disorder. Epilepsy does not necessarily "handicap" a person, but language, attitudes, and particular behaviors can. Educators and others must be particularly sensitive and considerate in these areas.

ADVANCES AND ALTERNATIVES

The educator should keep aware of the many changes occurring in the treatment and care of individuals with epilepsy. This awareness is particularly important if a student in your class or school is receiving a certain treatment or alternative type care. The newspaper from the Epilepsy Foundation of America (see "Resource") is an excellent resource for educators who wish to keep abreast of current advances in this field. Additionally, educators can obtain literature pertaining to a particular type of treatment or style of care by contacting the National Epilepsy Library (see "Resource") and through purchasing current educational products dealing with epilepsy (see "Resource").

The ketogenic diet and vagus nerve stimulation are examples of advances and alternatives the educator needs to be informed about. There are many more changes and new information being presented. However, the ketogenic diet and the vagus nerve stimulation can serve as models of advances and alternatives.

An alternative treatment for seizures is the ketogenic diet, a food regimen that is high in fat and low in carbohydrates. The diet creates a condition that makes the body metabolize body fat and generate a chemical termed ketones. When a sufficient amount of ketones are in the blood, seizures may be less in number or be eliminated. The exact reason for this condition affecting seizures is not fully understood, although it is now being recognized as a useful form of therapy (Schwartz, Boyes, & Aynsley-Green, 1989). According to an article on the ketogenic diet (Birch, March 30, 1993), "It appears to work because of a quirk in the chemistry of the body. Eating mostly fatty foods, it seems, has some of the same effects on the body as starvation" (p. 8a). It was noted that in biblical times fasting often reduced or stopped seizures (but the seizures reappeared when the fast was stopped).

There has been a renewed interest in this form of therapy. For example, Schwartz, Eaton, Bower, and Aynsley-Green (1989) found that the diet reduced seizure frequency, but noted that it can be quite unpalatable along with occurrences of diarrhea and vomiting. However, the authors noted that the diet was tolerated by children under the age of 15 years old. In addition, success has been reported using the diet with individuals with neurologic disabilities and intractable seizures (Kinsman, Vining, Quaskey, Mellits, & Freeman, 1992). The diet cannot be tried or experimented with at home. The food intake must be devised and supervised by a medical doctor trained in the regimen. The difficulty in having a student maintain such a diet, both at home and in school, is obvious.*

Most students with epilepsy control their seizures with antiepileptic

*Further information about this diet can be found in a book by John M. Freeman and Millicent T. Kelly, *The Epilepsy Diet Treatment* (New York: Demos Publications).

drugs. When this strategy is less than successful, brain surgery may be considered. However, such surgery is not always an alternative that can be taken by all individuals.

An alternative therapy currently under investigation is the Neuro-Cybernetic Prosthesis (NCP) system. At the present time, the system is being used with adults for the treatment of intractable complex partial seizures. A pacemaker type generator is implanted in the chest and is attached to the vagus nerve within the neck of the individual. Stimulation of the vagus nerve, which goes to and from the brain, is aimed at normalizing the brain waves. According to the patient information packet from Cyberonics (Webster, Texas), the company responsible for the device, a magnet is used to manually turn on the generator, in addition to the automatic stimulation delivered by the device. The device can be programed by an IBM compatible personal computer using software developed by the company (Terry, Tarver, & Zabara, 1991).

Research into the effect on the vagus nerve has been conducted with success (Hammond, Uthman, Reid, & Wilder, 1992). Other initial testing is positive, with over 50 percent of the individuals showing a 50 percent reduction in seizures (Terry et al., 1991). It appears to be a safe and effective intervention, with adverse effects being minimal (Wilder, Uthman, & Hammond, 1991). Individuals with auras seemed to benefit the most, although others could find the system beneficial as well (Holder, Wernicke, & Tarver, 1992). Definite conclusions about the overall effectiveness of the system must wait for results of larger numbers of tests (Salinsky & Burchiel, 1993). In addition, approval from appropriate federal agencies is needed prior to use by other individuals.

Many other alternatives and advances are being discussed and analyzed. For example, alternatives to traditional care include the use of biofeedback, relaxation therapies, herbal remedies, nutrition, and acupuncture (Goldberg, 1991), as well as chiropractic manipulation. Many of these alternatives for the treatment of epilepsy have not been investigated and researched thoroughly. Further research is needed to justify and verify the use of these techniques.

RESOURCE:

Epilepsy U.S.A.

This publication from the Epilepsy Foundation of America reports on recent developments in the field of epilepsy. The newspaper (which comes free with membership in the organization) provides a variety of types of informative articles, commentary, and newsbriefs.

Epilepsy U.S.A.
Epilepsy Foundation of America
4351 Garden City Drive
Landover, Maryland 20785

RESOURCE:

The Epilepsy Foundation of America
Catalog Sales Department
4351 Garden City Drive
Landover, MD 20785

Phone: (301) 577-0100
FAX: (301) 577-9056

Videos, books, and guides about epilepsy can be purchased.

RESOURCE:

National Epilepsy Library
Phone: (800) EFA-4050

A free service for professionals which includes a comprehensive information base about epilepsy utilizing journal articles, books, papers, newsletters, reprints, and custom searches.

Chapter 4

LEGISLATION

Historically, public school education was viewed as a privilege. However, today all students have a right to a free and appropriate public education at no cost to the parents. The following legislative acts have provided the necessary foundation to allow for these rights of all students with disabilities.

PUBLIC LAW 93–112 THE REHABILITATION ACT OF 1973 SECTION 504

Section 504 of P.L. 93-112, the Rehabilitation Act of 1973 outlaws discriminatory practices toward individuals with disabilities. States receiving any type of federal financial assistance must comply with this legislation. It states that

> no otherwise qualified handicapped individual . . . shall, solely by reason of his/her handicap, be excluded from participation in, be denied the benefits of, or be subject to discrimination under any program or activity receiving federal financial assistance (29 U.S.C. 794).

The Section 504 regulation defines a handicapped person as:

> (1) . . . any person who (i) has a physical or mental impairment which substantially limits one or more life activities; (ii) has a record of such an impairment, or (iii) is regarded as having such an impairment . . . (2) (ii) Major life activities means functions such as caring for one's self performing manual tasks, walking, seeing, hearing, speaking, breathing, learning, and working (34 Code of Federal Regulations (CFR) Section 104.3(j), 1988).

Often referred to as the Bill of Rights for the Handicapped (Gearheart, Mullen, & Gearheart, 1993), this law has many implications for individuals with disabilities. Section 504's thrust is to stop discrimination against this population. The antidiscrimination portion of Section 504 addresses three types of behavior: exclusion, denial of benefits, and discrimination (Epilepsy Foundation of America, 1992b). The law addresses all persons with disabilities, regardless of age. The legislation also includes discrimination in services, transportation, facilities, support services, supplies, and educational opportunities.

Section 504 requires a free and appropriate public education (FAPE) for each student with a disability, regardless of the severity of the disability. Exclusion from programs, including nonacademic and extracurricular, cannot be made based on the disability.

When compared to other legislation, it can be seen that Section 504 does not name disabilities but it includes a number of other disorders, such as attention deficit disorder, homelessness, AIDS, and epilepsy. When a health condition interferes with a student's ability to become involved with school activities, the student can be considered, within Section 504, as having a physical disability. This designation does not mean the person cannot function or participate in school. It does mean, however, that educators may need to use modifications, be flexible, and adapt the learning environment for the individual.

Section 504 is overseen by the Office for Civil Rights of the Department of Education. Regional offices are located throughout the United States. For additional information, contact the resource shown below.

RESOURCE:

U.S. Department of Education
Office For Civil Rights
Washington, DC 20202-1328
Phone: (202) 205-8686

PUBLIC LAW 94–142 THE EDUCATION OF ALL HANDICAPPED CHILDREN ACT

Public Law 94-142, The Education Of All Handicapped Children Act, has had a tremendous effect on the education of students with disabilities and is considered to be one of the most significant pieces of educational legislation in this century. The law, passed in 1975, contains mandates about the way educators work with this population of students. The major components of the law include:

- A free, appropriate public education for all students with disabilities between the ages of 3 and 21.

- A requirement that students be educated in the least restrictive environment. In many instances, this means the regular classroom. The intent of the law is to encourage, whenever possible, education with students that have no disabilities.
- An individualized education program (IEP) be developed for each student with a disability. The IEP, based on the student's present level of functioning, includes the goals and objectives, materials to be used, services and who will provide them, amount of mainstreaming in to regular classrooms, and evaluation procedures.
- Rights of the student and parents/guardians regarding assessment and placement procedures must be given. Nondiscriminatory practices must be employed.
- Efforts must be made to identify all students with disabilities.
- Students with disabilities must receive an appropriate education at no cost to the parents/guardians.
- An impartial due process hearing is available if the parents/guardians disagree with any of the school's decisions about the child's education.
- Evaluation procedures must be carried out by a multidisciplinary team of professionals.
- Training must be given to educators and other personnel who are involved with students with disabilities.

The Individualized Education Program (IEP) is a written agreement concerning the child's needs and what the school intends to do about those identified needs. The IEP must contain:

- The student's present level of academic functioning;
- Annual instructional goals for the student;
- Short-term objectives that are related to the annual goals;
- The special education and related services that will be provided to the student;
- The extent the student will participate in the regular classroom;
- The anticipated amount of time for each of the services; and
- Plans for evaluation of the goals and objectives.

The development of the IEP should have information coming from the student's teacher, school district representative(s), the student (when appropriate) and the parent/guardian, and other individuals, such as those who may have specific knowledge about the person's epilepsy and other conditions. Individuals whose services may be needed can play an important role in diagnoses and determination of an appropriate educational program.

The United States Office of Education defined handicapped children as those who have been evaluated and found to have one or more of the conditions listed and need special education and related services: deaf, deaf-blind, mentally retarded, multihandicapped, orthopedically impaired, other health impaired, seriously emotionally disturbed, specific learning disabilities, speech impaired, and visually handicapped (U.S. Office of Education, 1977, p. 42478).

According to Best, Bigge, and Sirvis (1990), P.L. 94-142 separates physical handicaps into two areas: (1) children with orthopedic handicaps (problems with skeleton, joints, and muscles) and (2) children with health impairments that affect educational performance. The United States Office of Education (1977) stated that this would include "limited strength, vitality, or alertness due to chronic or acute health problems such as a heart condition, tuberculosis, rheumatic fever, nephritis, asthma, sickle cell anemia, hemophilia, epilepsy, lead poisoning, leukemia, or diabetes" (p. 42478).

PUBLIC LAW 99–457 THE AMENDMENTS TO THE EDUCATION OF ALL HANDICAPPED CHILDREN ACT

On October 8, 1986, P.L. 99-457, which amended sections of P.L. 94-142, was signed. This law extends the regulations found in P.L. 94-142 to students between the ages of three and five. In order to receive federal funds, every state must now provide special education and related services to three- to five-year-old children with disabilities. The legislation also provides financial incentives to the state to provide early intervention programs for infants and toddlers (birth through two years of age) who are suspected of having, or are at risk of developing, disabilities.

Within this law is a mandate for development of the individualized family service plan (IFSP). Similar to an IEP, it establishes the direction for the program. The IFSP focuses on the needs of the child and the family. The plan is evaluated once per year, but it also is examined with the family once every six months. The components of the IFSP are:

- Information on the child's current level of functioning in: physical

development, cognition, speech and language development, psychosocial development, and self-help skills;
- The family's strengths and needs;
- The goals for the child and family;
- The criteria, procedures, and timeliness;
- Early intervention services needed, including the methods, amount of time, and duration of services;
- Transition procedures from early intervention to preschool programs.

Part H of the amendments was passed by Congress in 1986. Federal program requirements and funds to assist states develop interdisciplinary early intervention programs for children from birth to age three were created. The services in the programs are aimed at children designated as developmentally disabled, developmentally delayed, or at risk for delays, as well as for the families of these children.

PUBLIC LAW 101–336 AMERICANS WITH DISABILITIES ACT

The Americans With Disabilities Act is civil rights legislation for persons with disabilities. The ADA (Americans With Disabilities Act) became law on July 26, 1990. It addresses protection from various forms of discrimination, similar to the guarantees given to individuals regarding race, national origin, gender, and religion. The Civil Rights Division of the U.S. Department of Justice stated that the law guarantees equal opportunity for individuals with disabilities in employment, public accommodations, transportation, state and local government services, and telecommunications. Many of the practices and accommodations are similar to Section 504 of the Rehabilitation Act. However, the ADA is not limited to discriminatory acts by agencies receiving federal funds, as Section 504 is.

The law defines a person with a disability as:

> (1) a person with a physical or mental impairment that substantially limits that person in some major life activity (such as walking, talking, breathing, or working); (2) a person with a record of such a physical or mental impairment (such as a person with a history of mental illness or heart disease who no longer has the disease, but who is discriminated against because of their record of an impairment); or (3) a person who is regarded as having such an impairment (such as a person who has a significant burn on his/her face which does not limit

him/her in any major life activity but who is discriminated against). (American with Disabilities Act, 1990, p. 1)

Among the major points of the law are:

- Employers with 15 or more employees cannot discriminate against persons with disabilities; accommodations must be made for persons with disabilities unless "undue hardship" can be shown;
- New construction and alterations to existing facilities must be accessible;
- Buses and rail transportation must be accessible;
- Public accommodations such as restaurants, hotels, day-care centers, parks, and doctors' offices cannot discriminate due to disability; and
- Telephone companies must have telecommunications relay services 24 hours per day for hearing-impaired and speech-impaired persons.

Most individuals with epilepsy do not need large numbers of accommodations in order to function successfully within the community. There are, however, suggested accommodations related to the workplace that may be considered for certain individuals with epilepsy. For example, the Epilepsy Foundation of America (1992b) suggested a number of types of changes:

- Job restructuring—i.e. redistributing nonessential, marginal job functions, such as driving, in cases where driving is not a central job requirement and may be performed by other employees.
- Replacing a flickering light in an employee's work area if the person's seizures are triggered by such flashing lights.
- Scheduling consistent work shifts to accommodate persons whose seizure activity is exacerbated by inconsistent sleep patterns.
- Allowing an employee who fatigues easily due to side effects of medication the opportunity to take more frequent breaks.
- Allowing an individual to work a flexible schedule to accommodate his/her seizure activity or need to see a doctor (p. 8).

Of particular importance is the fact that employers must make reasonable accommodations based on the employee's request. The intent is to help the employee manage job duties within one's capabilities. However, a person could be rejected from a job if the person presents a threat to the health or safety of him/herself or to others in the workplace. In addition, the person can lose the job if the job cannot be done satisfactorily after accommodations are made.

A major thrust of this legislation is to allow and encourage the integration of individuals with disabilities into mainstream society. For example, it is against the law to discriminate against a person because of a medical condition, such as epilepsy. The legislation also limits and guides pre-employment questions regarding medical conditions. It is against the law to refuse access to city parks and recreational facilities for a person with epilepsy (U.S. Dept. of Justice). Requirements that screen out individuals with disabilities (i.e. requiring a driver's license as the only means of identification) are also against the law. Individuals, including students with epilepsy, who will be seeking employment and transitioning to the world of work should be made aware of their rights and the provisions of this law. The Americans With Disabilities Act is, indeed, landmark legislation. The full impact of this legislation will continue to be felt in future years.

RESOURCE:

The Americans With Disabilities Act:
A Guide To Provisions Affecting Persons
With Epilepsy

E.F.A.
Catalogue Sales Dept.
4351 Garden City Drive
Landover, MD 20785-2267
Phone: (301) 577-0100

RESOURCE:

For additional information, contact:
Office on the Americans with Disability Act
Civil Rights Division
P.O. Box 66118
Washington D.C. 20035-6118

(202) 514-0301 (voice)
(202) 514-0383 (TDD)
(202) 514-6193 (Electronic Bulletin Board)

RESOURCE:

U.S. Architectural & Transportation Compliance Board
1111 18th St. N.W.

Suite 501
Washington, D.C. 20036
Phone: (800) USA-ABLE

RESOURCE:

For Legal Action:
Equal Employment Opportunity Commission
Phone: (800) 669-4000

RESOURCE:

For information on accommodation strategies:
Job Accommodation Network
West Virginia University
Morgantown, WV
Phone: (800) 526-7234 or (800) 232-9675

PUBLIC LAW 101–392 THE CARL D. PERKINS VOCATIONAL AND APPLIED TECHNOLOGY EDUCATION ACT AMENDMENTS OF 1990

This legislation was signed into law on September 25, 1990. The law amended the original Carl D. Perkins Act, which provided funds for vocational education programs, including those students with disabilities. Closely related to the Individuals With Disabilities Education Act (P.L. 101-476), it extends the guarantees of vocational education opportunities for students with disabilities.

PUBLIC LAW 101–476 THE INDIVIDUALS WITH DISABILITIES EDUCATION ACT

Public Law 101-476, The Individuals With Disabilities Act (IDEA), passed in 1990, extends the components of P.L. 94-142. The law includes the following:

- Autism and traumatic brain injury (TBI) were added to the list of disabilities;
- Transition services from school to postschool activities must be written into the IEP or ITP (individualized transition plan); these

plans must be written no later than when the student is sixteen years old;

- Related services now include rehabilitation counseling, assistive technology services, recreational therapy, and social work services. These services are in addition to those already stated in P.L. 94-142.
- There is more emphasis on education in the least restrictive environment (LRE) and promoting the integration of students with disabilities into regular classrooms;
- The language in the law has changed from using "handicapped children" to "children with disabilities";
- States may be sued in federal courts when violations of the law occur.

Within this law (IDEA), transition services for special education students are required. The vocational training plan within the IEP (or written as the ITP) must be devised by the time the student is sixteen years old. Many school districts have started the ITP phase at a much earlier age.

The ITP is a written plan to guide the student between school and postschool activities. It focuses on educational programs, vocational placements, work settings, and independent living. The ITP includes annual goals, short-term objectives associated with the skills needed to function in the community and on the job, transitional services needed and other plans for the student for successful transition. In many cases the ITP can be a part of the IEP.

RESOURCE:

DISABILITY RIGHTS AND WRONGS by Keren Marder

A quarterly report of current court cases; descriptions of issues written for the general public; FREE.

Contact:
EFA Legal Advocacy Dept.
4351 Garden City Drive
Landover, MD 20785
Phone: (301) 459-3700

IMPLICATIONS FOR THE EDUCATION OF STUDENTS WITH EPILEPSY

What are the educational implications of this legislation for a student with epilepsy? Under P.L. 94-142 and P.L. 101-476's definition of children with disabilities, students with epilepsy are among those who are eligible to receive special education services under the category of "other health impairments." Students may have an additional disorder, such as learning disabilities, autism, traumatic brain injury, or mental retardation that they possess concurrently. Having epilepsy, however, does not automatically allow a student to receive special services. *School district procedures must be followed in order to determine eligibility and the disorder must affect the student's performance in school to the degree that special education and/or related services are needed.* The Epilepsy Foundation of America (1992b) stated that a student "who is experiencing learning difficulties associated with his or her seizure condition is entitled to special education and related services, even if the seizure condition is the sole medical condition" (p. 24). It is important to remember that criteria for various special education services vary from region to region.

State education departments establish guidelines and requirements as reflected by the disability stated within the laws. States are required to implement the mandates derived from federal laws. State laws must be in accordance with federal regulations, even though the state may vary or even go beyond the federal regulations. The federal guidelines give the state flexibility in implementing the laws. Each state has its own regulations for special needs services, as well as state plans regarding the means to providing a free, appropriate education for students with disabilities. The State Education Department can provide a copy of the state's special education regulations, as well as the guidelines for its implementation.

Individuals also have a right to examine local school district plans for educating students with special needs. These written plans must be in line with the state plan for the education of this population of students. School district administrators can provide the appropriate procedures for obtaining the local school district plan.

Other implications from this past legislation for the education of students with epilepsy include the following:

- The students, including those with disabilities, are entitled to a free, appropriate, public education in the least restrictive environment;

often, this means the person will be educated with other students without disabilities;

- Exclusion from academic, nonacademic, and extracurricular programs cannot be made due to epilepsy; however, safety factors can and should be considered;
- Discrimination is against the law; students with epilepsy are entitled to comparable education, services, and support;
- Students are entitled to be considered for obtaining related services;
- Parents and professionals have a right to due process procedures with respect to identification, evaluation, or program placement;
- Students are entitled to a multidisciplinary and nondiscriminatory evaluation;
- Services are available for children from birth to twenty-one years of age;
- Students with disabilities must have a school transition plan written prior to sixteen years of age;
- Students with epilepsy will have access to more normalized experiences in our schools, with inclusion, integration, and independence playing a major role.

Laws have very little effect until courts derive interpretations and meaning from them. Suits will be filed and the subsequent decisions may clarify the various legislative acts. Indeed, future legal cases will expand our knowledge concerning the rights of all students to receive an appropriate education.

Chapter 5

SCHOOL AND THE STUDENT WITH EPILEPSY

Many students with epilepsy do well in school. There is no reason to believe that epilepsy goes hand in hand with learning and social/emotional problems. Although problems in these areas occur more frequently in students with epilepsy, it is inaccurate to make generalized assumptions.

Most students with epilepsy remain in the regular classroom. Significant differences between students with and without epilepsy in intelligence and achievement do not exist. Some students may need special education services and others do not. Each student must be viewed as an individual; and educational programs, related services, program adjustments and modifications are developed and implemented based on the individual's particular needs. The relationship between regular education and special education with respect to educating students with chronic conditions was stated appropriately by Lynch et al. (1992):

> The strengths and weaknesses of current regular and special education systems, the range of educational options that students with chronic illnesses need, and the flexibility and rapid response time that is required for students with some chronic illnesses suggest that a coordinated partnership between regular and special education programs and services presents the best approach to service delivery. Such a proposal is in keeping with the philosophy that all students should begin with the regular classroom environment, adding only those supports that are needed; and it affirms that students with chronic illnesses are the responsibility of the entire school. (p. 218)

There are a number of factors to consider in order to determine the reason a particular student may have a problem in school. Intelligence, motivation, behavior, learning abilities, etc., only begin the list of potential influences. Learning problems are more common with this population, but one should also remember that there are many other students without epilepsy that have problems in school (Freeman et al., 1990).

Educators can assist the student to cope with and adjust to the disorder. School personnel must recognize and understand epilepsy in order to help others. However, educators are often prevented from providing appropriate interventions for this population due to a lack of accurate information, proper management procedures, and knowledge of associated disorders (Dreisbach et al., 1982).

Communication among families, health care providers, and educators must be ongoing. Emergency planning is necessary, recognizing that educators must know the particulars of an emergency situation and the various symptoms and signals related to it. In addition, it must be recognized that some students with chronic conditions have numerous school absences that affect school performance.

Many students with epilepsy have some degree of control over their seizures by the use of medication, others do not. Some individuals may even be able to taper off the medication (under medical supervision) and be seizure free. However, no one can predict when a seizure can or will occur. Fear, anxiety, and uncertainty often prevail with those individuals involved with the student.

FROM THE CLASSROOM:

> [A school nurse states . . .] **"This is still a condition that we don't talk about. Everyone is concerned with Lyme disease, asthma, Reye's syndrome, rabies, etc., and we don't talk about seizure disorders."**

THE ROLE OF THE EDUCATOR

What are the various roles and functions of the educator to help a student with epilepsy and the family within the context of the school environment?

The educator can:

- Assist in the identification of students with seizures;
- Help the student understand epilepsy and seizures;
- Help the family understand epilepsy and seizures;
- Act as a resource for the family;
- Provide direct assistance to the student for the physical management of the disorder;
- Assist the student in coping with the disorder;
- Help the student to become an integral member of the classroom and school;

- Help dispel myths, prejudices, and misinformation concerning the disorder;
- Implement first-aid procedures;
- Provide assistance if learning and/or behavior difficulties result from the disorder and/or medication effects;
- Play an active part in the school community that creates a viable, appropriate educational program for the student;
- Refer the student, if needed, for special help;
- Assist the student and family in obtaining support services;
- Be a part of the student's support system;
- Help implement the individualized adaptations needed by the student;
- Be an active advocate for the student and family;
- Utilize strategies that develop the student's self-esteem;
- Play a major role in helping to create a more normalized school life for the student;
- Teach other students about epilepsy and seizures;
- Educate colleagues and other professionals about epilepsy and seizures;
- Help the student develop personal strengths and talents; and
- Treat the student as a person, not as a disability.

In order for an educator to assume any of these roles, a proactive stance must be taken. Some essential questions to assist the educator in beginning to address these particular areas are given:

Who are the key people in your area that are concerned with health and the schools?

Who are the educational leaders in your area who are making significant decisions about students with special needs?

What supports and resources exist in your area for the student with epilepsy?

Who has experience and training in dealing with students with epilepsy?

Going beyond these first questions, the educator can begin to establish a more detailed plan of action. The following information can assist the educator in this endeavor.

SOME PRELIMINARY QUESTIONS

If the educator knows in advance that a student with epilepsy will be in the classroom, there is an opportunity to obtain some basic information about the specific condition. By talking with medical personnel, such as the student's doctor, school nurse, etc., and the parents/guardian, vital information can be obtained. There is a need to establish a connection among family, school, and medical personnel in order to provide quality services (Dreisbach et al., 1982). A preliminary set of questions could include:

- What type of seizure does the person have?
- How long does the seizure last?
- What is seen when the person has a seizure?
- Does the person experience any aura or exhibit any particular behaviors prior to the seizure?
- How does the person behave and feel after a seizure?
- How often does the person have a seizure?
- When was the last seizure?
- What medication does the person take and how often is it taken?
- What type of emergency care would you as the parent/guardian like taken during and after the seizure?
- Under what conditions do you as the parents/guardians want to be notified?
- What other concerns do you have for your child within the school environment?
- As parents/guardians, what concerns do you have with the school policy on medical emergencies, medication guidelines, school nurse's procedures, etc.?

THE NEED FOR SPECIAL ASSISTANCE

Students with epilepsy can find the effects of the disorder range on a continuum of a mild inconvenience to a severe developmental disorder. It must be determined to what degree the disorder interferes with learning, achievement, and other school functions. Epilepsy may exist in combination with other impairments, such as mental retardation, emotional disabilities, autism, and cerebral palsy. To address the need for assistance, some questions for consideration are posed:

- To what degree does the disorder interfere with the student's learning and achievement in school?
- To what degree does the anticonvulsant medication interfere with the student's learning and achievement in school?

- How often has the student missed school due to the disorder?
- To what degree has the student been affected socially/emotionally from the stigma associated with the disorder?
- Does the student have any documented learning disabilities?
- Does the student have any other impairments, such as mental retardation, autism, cerebral palsy, or multiple disabilities?
- Are the seizures under control? What is the frequency and duration of the seizures?
- What is the student's level of self-esteem and emotional ability?
- What are the student's other health needs?
- To what degree can the student function successfully in the regular classroom?

After such informal considerations, a more formal approach is necessary. Assessment procedures play a major role in determining the learning environment, special services, and program modifications needed by the student. A thorough assessment of all facets of the student's strengths and weaknesses must be conducted. Too often in the past an oversimplified concept of epilepsy by educators existed (Dreisbach et al., 1982).

ASSESSMENT

The process of assessment is an important element in education. It determines a student's strengths and weaknesses and allows educators to make sound decisions. Educators may use the assessment process to obtain data for program screening, program evaluation, current levels of functioning of a student, special education placement, and IEP plans. Assessment is a vital and integral part of the educational process.

ASSESSMENT CONSIDERATIONS

There are a number of important considerations before implementing assessments with a student with epilepsy. First, consider anxiety and stress levels. All students experience a degree of anxiety in the testing situation; however, this population of students may experience particular difficulty when under severe stress. Second, the health of the student at the time of test taking must be considered. The student should be performing at the usual pace and in the usual manner at the time of assessment. If the student has had a seizure recently or is not working at the usual pace for whatever reason, the usefulness of the results will be limited. Third, some students may need testing modifications in order to obtain an accurate picture of the strengths and weaknesses. The modifications need to be stated on the IEP and can include such adaptations as:

- paraphrased instructions,
- extended time limits,
- use of aids, such as a calculator,
- test location could be changed, such as to a comfortable room instead of the testing room, and
- use of praise

THE EVALUATION

If the student needs additional help or is having problems in school, an evaluation to determine the specific problems is warranted. The evaluation team may be known by different names, such as the Child Study Team, Committee on Special Education, Pupil Evaluation Team, Multidisciplinary Team, etc.

The school district typically utilizes specialists, when needed, for particular components of the IEP. For example, a learning disabilities specialist, psychologist, school nurse, physician, etc., might be used in conducting an evaluation. The evaluation process might also include interviews with the parent and child, a physical examination, medical records, etc.

Although there have not been educational tests developed for use only with persons with epilepsy, an epilepsy stressor inventory (ESI) was created to help individuals with epilepsy identify stress factors in their lives. Respondents first indicate on a 4-point Lickert type scale the extent of experiencing stress for each stress factor from "never" to "frequently a problem." Sample items include: "Uncertainty about when a seizure will occur; Overprotection by family or friends; Need to take medication regularly," etc. (p. 11). If a factor is identified as a stressor, a 3-point Likert type scale is used to rate each stressor, ranging from "little stress" to "much stress." Twenty-two stressor items were used with subjects who ranged in age from 18 to 65 years old in the revised epilepsy stressor inventory (Snyder, 1993). School personnel may find this tool useful for students who are 18 years of age and older.

Educators must remember that no single assessment procedure can be used as the criterion for establishing the educational program for a student. Regulations mandate that various sources of information from a number of people be obtained and the subsequent program be developed based on the needs of the particular student.

NEUROPSYCHOLOGICAL ASSESSMENT

Neuropsychological assessment is a highly recommended process to use in the evaluation of students with epilepsy. It is a broad evaluation of cognitive abilities and skills. The assessment is "generally viewed as the administration and interpretation of a set of psychometric tests measuring a broad range of specific cognitive abilities required for success at school and community" (Ewing-Cobbs & Fletcher, 1990, pp. 111–112). The abilities being examined include general cognition, language, visual perception, attention, concentration, learning ability, memory, motor, and psychological functions. In addition to standardized test results, other factors, such as motivation, emotional status and central nervous system dysfunction inferences, can be made (Ewing-Cobbs & Fletcher, 1990). The comprehensive evaluation also includes historical information on the student, neuro-medical findings, observations from interviews and testing situations, and psychological adjustment (Collum, Kuck, & Ruff, 1990). The results may offer information about the student's abilities/disabilities regarding information processing skills (Smith, 1991).

Neuropsychologists may opt to use neuropsychological test batteries or use traditional tests supplemented with other assessments of specific abilities. The interpretation of the results include which brain areas stand for the strengths and weaknesses (Smith, 1991). Cognitive measures can also be used to measure certain abilities, such as attention and memory (Ewing-Cobbs & Fletcher, 1990). Although approaches to assessment may differ, there are some commonalities. According to Ewing-Cobbs and Fletcher (1990), each approach to neuropsychological assessment includes:

- a definition of the problem;
- identification of other cognitive skills associated with the problem;

- specifying environmental and cultural factors which could affect test performance;
- information is combined with biological and medical sources with respect to central nervous system; and
- the remedial plan is based on assessment data.

In a more general sense, the use of a neuropsychological approach suggests a relationship, as well as a causal association, between the brain and behavior (Obrznt & Hynd, 1990). Neuropsychology examines specific learning abilities that are related to brain function, a particularly important aspect for students with epilepsy.

GUIDELINES FOR BEST PRACTICES WITH STUDENTS WITH EPILEPSY

The purpose of establishing a set of guidelines for educators is to help promote sound practices, clear directions, and appropriate programs. A philosophy and set of values can be used as a framework for program development and educational interventions. In addition, such information can be used to generate "best practices" for a given field.

A foundation for the beliefs and ideas offered here is that all students with epilepsy should be given the opportunities presented to all students. Rights and needs are to be addressed, as well as the development of subsequent educational interventions and programs. The student with epilepsy has a right to develop potential to the fullest.

The following statements are presented as beginning steps in establishing guidelines for educating this population of students. The list is not complete or inclusive, and educators are encouraged to add their own beliefs, practices, and ideas to it:

- The students have a wide range of abilities; some students may need special considerations and assistance and others may not;
- Students with epilepsy do not necessarily have a disability; some students will experience a mild inconvenience while others will be legally disabled;
- Students should attend their regular neighborhood school with their peers, no matter what other disabilities the person might have;
- Students should enroll in classes that reflect their individual strengths and limitations; epilepsy itself is not a determinant of program;

- Students and their families have a right to make choices and to have control over decisions that will affect their education;
- Students have a right to a free, appropriate education and related services, if deemed necessary by the school district's committee on special education;
- Students should have a right not to be discriminated against and to participate in schools without stigma associations;
- Students and their families have a right to full and unconditional support from all members of the educational community (i.e. administrators, teachers, paraprofessionals, school bus drivers, custodians, etc.);
- Students should have the right to participate in extracurricular and recreational school activities with all other students; restrictions and safety measures should be made on an individual basis;
- See the child as a total student, not as epilepsy or a seizure disorder only;
- Be careful about being overprotective; avoid treating students with epilepsy with extreme caution;
- Talk directly and honestly to the student with epilepsy; obtain the concerns, interests, fears, etc., of the student; have the family become comfortable talking to you about their feelings concerning epilepsy;
- Teach the student personal responsibility; such responsibility leads to a sense of personal control;
- Develop a strong relationship with the school nurse; this person plays a vital role in the lives of students with epilepsy;
- The educational program for a student with epilepsy should be created around the needs of the individual; for example, consideration of the classroom schedule and optimum learning times should be viewed; the medication effects, seizure occurrence, and times of seizures should influence scheduling and learning opportunities;
- Relax—Students with epilepsy are more like other children than they are different.

FROM THE CLASSROOM:

[A teacher states . . .] **"The staff has been excellent. They are calm and reassuring to the child. Classmates express concern for the student's well-being after seizures occur. Most of the time we are able to have the child resume**

> **his class work. Occasionally he must be taken from the classroom to rest."**
>
> **[A school nurse states . . .] "Many times she [student] announces to the class that the seizure is coming, but by the time I can be notified by the teacher, the seizure is over and she is back at work in the class."**

MODIFICATIONS

In order to address the varied needs of this population of students within the placement options, modifications of the environment may be necessary. The following adaptations may be useful in developing an appropriate program based on a child's individual needs:

- Permit unscheduled rest periods if needed;
- Reduce subject/work load due to rest and recovery periods; this may be quickly increased at a later point when it has been determined that the child is ready;
- Consider medication effects when dealing with the school schedule; for example, the more difficult work could be given in the morning when the child is least affected by the medication (or vice versa);
- Provide resource room assistance, special education services, and/or related services if needed;
- Allow unrestricted access to the school nurse's office;
- Use an itinerant teacher in the home if the student is out of school for large amounts of time;
- Provide peer assistance when needed;
- Direct the student to counseling/discussions with the school counselor, if needed;
- Obtain adapted physical education, if necessary;
- Maintain communication with the child if hospitalized;
- Use oral testing or varied testing formats if the student is designated as learning disabled or has another condition that interferes with learning;
- Provide for varied arrangements for school events that are stressful (i.e. lengthy tests) for students who have increased the chance of experiencing a seizure due to stress.

- If school absences due to seizures are a problem, allow the student opportunities to make up the work;
- If school tardiness due to morning seizures is a problem, create adaptions which allow the student the time to make up the work;
- Treat the student fairly; Hallahan and Kauffman (1994) noted that students in the classroom often learn how to act with individuals with disabilities by watching the teacher.

For the benefit of the student, the educator must take the initiative to maintain a communication link among the family, school, and medical personnel.

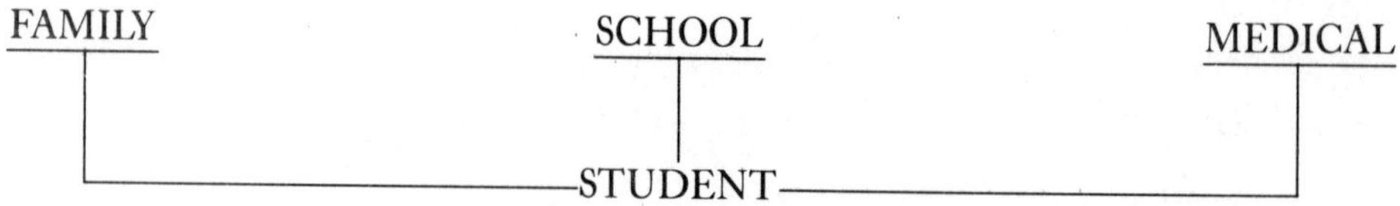

Figure 2. The Communication Link

ADDITIONAL SERVICES

The educational needs of students with epilepsy are becoming more clearly defined. Educators are responding to the learning needs of this population of students within the classroom. Other services also may be needed to meet the demands of students with epilepsy. Legislative acts have responded to students who are recognized as having a disability by addressing issues such as additional, or related, services.

Public Law 94-142 requires related services be provided to students with disabilities, when needed and stated on the Individualized Education Program. Related services means:

> transportation and such developmental, corrective, and other supportive services as are required to assist a handicapped child to benefit from special education, and includes speech pathology and audiology, psychological services, physical and occupational therapy, recreation, early identification and assessment of disabilities in children, counseling services, and medical services for diagnostic and evaluation purposes. The term also includes school health services, social work services in schools, and parent counseling and training (United States Office Of Education, 1977, p. 42479).

It is the school's responsibility to establish and provide the needed related services. When a service is stated in the IEP, it will be provided at no cost to the family.

Public Law 94-142 stated thirteen related services that students with disabilities may obtain in their special education programs:

- audiology
- occupational therapy
- physical therapy
- psychological services
- medical services for diagnostic or evaluative purposes only
- school health services
- counseling services
- speech-language pathology
- social work services
- parent counseling and training
- recreation therapy
- early identification and assessment of disabilities in children (34 Code of Federal Regulations (CFR) Section 300.13 (b)(1)–(13), 1988).

The Individuals With Disabilities Education Act (IDEA) defined "related services" as:

> . . . transportation, and such developmental, corrective, and other supportive services (including speech pathology and audiology, psychological services, physical and occupational therapy, recreation, including therapeutic recreation and social work services, and medical and counseling services, including rehabilitation counseling, except that such medical services shall be for diagnostic and evaluation purposes only) as may be required to assist a child with a disability to benefit from special education. (20 U.S.C. Chapter 33, Section 1401 (17), 1991)

A number of services may have to be delivered to students with disabilities in order to provide an appropriate education. In addition to those listed here, there may be other services which a student may need, such as assistive technology devices and services. In addition to the federal listing of services, states may include other related services in their regulations. For example, the National Information Center for Children and Youth With Disabilities (1991) noted that some states have included mobility training, dance therapy, and artistic and cultural programs as related services.

A number of court cases have resulted in information about school districts' responsibility for providing types of medical services within the category or related services. These cases have relevance to educators concerned with students with epilepsy, as well as other health disorders.

Some medically related services must be provided by the schools, as stated in *Irving Independent School District* v. *Tatro* (1979). This court case ruled that catheterization was a related service and that in order for a student to obtain a free and appropriate education, the procedure must be provided by the school district.

In the case of *Detsel* v. *Board of Education of Auburn Enlarged City School District* (1986), the court stated that a school district does not have to provide continuous nursing care for a student with a physical disability. Since the care was needed for maintenance of the student's life and the expertise needed was beyond the training of a school nurse, the conclusion was that the care was not a related service but was medical treatment.

The student with epilepsy may need help with taking medications, and the teacher, as well as other school personnel, may need specific training in first-aid procedures. These accommodations may be necessary for the student to receive an appropriate education. "The Epilepsy Foundation of America believes that both of these activities should be regarded as related services and as supportive services which permit the child to remain in school" (Epilepsy Foundation of America, 1992b, p. 25).

In a survey conducted by the California State Council on Developmental Disabilities (1992), it was found that students with seizure disorders had difficulties in keeping up with schoolwork because of medication side effects and school absenteeism. One of the results of the survey was that tutoring was a major support service needed by this population of students.

One of the problem areas, however, has been that in order to benefit from these laws that mandate related services, the student had to be identified as being a special education student. Students with epilepsy may or may not be designated as enrolled in special education. In order for a student to receive services and enroll in programs, the guidelines discussed for the Rehabilitation Act of 1973 would have to be used. "Section 504 (of the Rehabilitation Act) does not require a student to be enrolled in special education in order to receive related services" (National Information Center, 1991, p. 8). After a student is recognized as having a disability within the context of Section 504, schools must provide a free, appropriate education with related services to that student "without regard to the nature or severity of the individual's disability" (National Information Center, 1991, p. 9). School districts must comply with these regulations in order to maintain Federal financial assistance to the school district.

THE SCHOOL NURSE

All education personnel need to work collaboratively with the parents to address the issues related to disabilities (Santilli et al., 1991). Since the passage of the Education of All Handicapped Children Act of 1975, many students with disabilities have been integrated into the public school system. Many of these students have health problems that have caused school nurses to deal with new issues (Frank, 1990).

The school nurse is in a key position to manage chronically ill students in the school system (Joachim, 1989) and to offer accurate information about epilepsy to school personnel (Santilli et al., 1991). In fact, it has been suggested that the disorder of epilepsy could be used as an example within an educational model to teach health professionals about chronic conditions (Buchanan & Scambler, 1993).

School nurses have been involved with educating individuals in the schools about seizure disorders, even though they have had little exposure to children with epilepsy in their nursing education programs and may have had no on-the-job training for this work (Frank, 1990). They also need to be involved with the total collaborative effort by working with the educators, other medical personnel, and parents in addressing the total needs of the students with epilepsy.

A school-based project (Hazelnis, 1991) was conducted to identify the issues and concerns of public school nurses concerning students with seizure disorders in the schools. Thirty-seven school nurses responded to the survey by identifying issues of concern. In order of importance, issues were the education of the staff (30%), safety of the child (20%), education of peers (17%), development of the child's self-esteem (13%), communication between parents and school (11%), medication regime (6%), and first-aid procedures (3%) (Hazelnis, 1991).*

*An excellent resource for further reading on the roles and functions of the school nurse with respect to the student with epilepsy is Santilli, N., Dodson, W. E., & Walton, A. V. (1991), *Students with seizures: A manual for school nurses* (New Jersey: HealthScan).

RESOURCE:

National Association of School Nurses
Lamplighter Lane
P.O. Box 1300
Scarborough, Maine 04070-1300
Phone: (207) 883-2117

RESOURCE:

NICHCY
NATIONAL INFORMATION CENTER FOR CHILDREN AND YOUTH WITH DISABILITIES
P.O. Box 1492
Washington, D.C. 20013-1492
Phone: (703) 893-6061
Toll-free: (800) 999-5599
TDD: (703) 893-8614

NICHCY provides free information to individuals working with persons with disabilities; services include personal responses to questions, referrals to other organizations, publications, guides, and fact sheets, as well as providing technical assistance.

SUBSTITUTE TEACHERS

One of the more difficult jobs in education may be that of the substitute teacher. This person must often come into an unfamiliar classroom at a moment's notice, quickly obtain the teacher's plan for the day, and carry out the educational program with students that are unfamiliar.

It is extremely important that the substitute teacher be made aware of the health conditions of all the students in the classroom. Often this is accomplished through an attachment of a student's special conditions in the teacher's planbook. Substitute teachers must take the time to review this listing prior to the beginning of the day. The regular classroom teacher should note in this attachment any special procedures or considerations to be followed with particular students with special needs.

THE INDIVIDUALIZED HEALTH CARE PLAN

In order to provide an appropriate education for students with special health conditions, the impact of health conditions on a student's functioning in school must be addressed. Each state creates its own health screening criteria and programs for students. Evaluations and Individualized Education Programs (IEP) should include health information that can be derived from multidisciplinary assessments conducted by health personnel. The health and emergency needs of the student must be addressed in order to have the student function in the school environment.

Standards for practice have been established by various organizations, including the National Association of School Nurses. These standards were created to help guide the school nurse in the work done in schools. One of the accepted standards is the "development of individualized health (care) plans" (American Federation of Teachers, 1992). The Individualized Health Care Plan (IHCP) should include:

(a) the medical diagnosis
(b) symptoms and signals of danger or concern related to the medical condition
(c) medical treatments being received by the student and the schedule of treatments
(d) medications being received by the student, including type of medication, schedule, and possible side effects
(e) dietary needs of the student
(f) special equipment and supplies, if needed
(g) an overview of the family concerns
(h) an assessment of the social concerns related to the student
(i) written goals and objectives as well as who is responsible for each aspect of the IHCP
(j) school and classroom modifications needed
(k) safety procedures and emergency plans to be followed
(l) level of student independence
(m) dates of implementation and review procedures

The IHCP procedure should be started by having the school nurse, or other health professional, obtain the necessary background information on the student with special health needs. This person should then complete the necessary school nurse assessment.

Goals and objectives are identified for the student. Interventions that must take place in the school are established, as well as who will be in charge of the procedures. The needed training, and who will conduct it, must be established. Medication(s) and guidelines for the administration must be stated. Other areas of concern for the IHCP include the student's diet, special transportation procedures, classroom and school modifications needed, appropriate special equipment and supplies, safety procedures and emergency plans to be followed, degree of student independence and amount of assistance needed. Dates of implementation and review procedures should be stated with appropriate signatures. The parent(s), school nurse, school administrator, student's teacher, and designated others should act as a team to formulate this plan.

School health services are considered to be a related service and are part of the process of establishing an IEP, if the student is designated as being in need of special education services. Thus, the Individualized Health Care Plan (IHCP) may be part of the Individualized Education Program (IEP) if the student is enrolled in a special education program. Otherwise, if there is no IEP, the necessary medical information discussed would be included on the IHCP.

The process described can be seen as the following:

(1) School nurse/medical assessment is conducted
(2) Health care plan is established
(3) Health service plan created
(4) If the student has a disability, the health plan is incorporated into the IEP.
(5) If student does not have a disability, the health plan is incorporated into the IHCP.

School nurses are working more closely with the special education staff in the identification, assessment, evaluation, and development of the Individualized Education Program (IEP). Specific needs of the student are stated and how those needs will be met are outlined on the IEP. With such procedures established, this health care plan becomes an important component of the student's overall school program.

Be sure to familiarize yourself with the school district's or agency's procedures for dealing with confidential information. The record keeping for the administration of medication, the health care administration sheet, and the seizure events documentation log are examples of confidential information.

EXTRACURRICULAR ACTIVITIES

Participation in extracurricular activities plays an important part in schooling. The benefits to all students are numerous, such as learning to participate with others, cooperation, and heightened self-esteem. All students should have these activities as part of their school life. No one should be denied an opportunity to join and participate in after-school activities, in school intramural sports, clubs, etc. In fact, a strong argument could be made for why it is particularly important for students with epilepsy to participate with their peer group in both individual and group events.

SPORTS

Freeman, Vining, and Pillas (1990) take an individualized and commonsense approach to sports participation by students with epilepsy. The authors noted that "no blanket statement about sports participation for persons with epilepsy is possible" (p. 250) and all factors about the person, such as type of seizure, degree of control, etc., and the particular risks and protections for the sport must be taken into consideration. With these safeguards in mind, Anspaugh, Gilliland, and Anspaugh (1980) stated that the student with epilepsy "must be made to feel that they can participate in all facets of school life, including physical activities, team sports, and athletic contests" (p. 38GE). In fact, there is more of a chance of negative psychological effects from not being allowed to participate in athletics than having the risk of a seizure during an activity (Rowland, 1990).

Gates (1991) presented some factors which should be taken into consideration when an individual with epilepsy is considering participating in a sport. The author states that the greatest risk is when there is the possibility of falling and the participation in contact and water sports. Activities which may require special considerations include rope climbing, horseback riding, using the parallel bars, and jumping on the trampoline. The American Academy of Pediatrics (1983) also lists high diving and competitive underwater swimming as activities that should be avoided. Head protection was noted to be an important consideration for all students. In addition, Gates (1991) stressed the importance of contacting the student's neurologist regarding any participation in heavy contact sports. The responsibility for making the final decisions about participation in particular activities should be shared by the parents, physician, and the student (American Academy of Pediatrics, 1983).

Swimming

A student with epilepsy should not be alone in the water. Unsupervised swimming and swimming in open waterways should not be allowed (Kemp & Sibert, 1993). Everyone involved with the student should be aware of the condition and what should be done if a seizure occurs. No matter what type of seizure the student has, it is usually best to proceed with caution. A child with epilepsy is 7.5 times more apt to have an incident in water than a child without epilepsy (Kemp & Sibert, 1993). However, students with epilepsy who are supervised in water do not, according to these authors, have a greater chance of drowning than the regular population. Children with mental retardation and epilepsy, though, are "more prone to all types of accidental trauma" (Kemp & Sibert, 1993, p. 685).

If a seizure occurs when the student is in water, the person's head should be supported and moved to the side. Check for breathing and perform artificial respiration if it is necessary. Medical care may be needed if water was taken in.

FROM THE CLASSROOM:

> **[A school nurse states . . .] "We had a student fall during gym. He convulsed and another student recognized it as a seizure. He got the gym teacher and notified the school nurse."**

Driver Education

All information about the student and the particular type of epilepsy should be taken into consideration before a decision about driving an automobile is made. Although adults with epilepsy have been found to be at a higher risk for accident and traffic violations compared to the general public (Hansotia & Broste, 1993), it is important not to make generalizations about students with epilepsy and driving. Each case must be treated individually, examining the risks and benefits of driving to the person and society (Ozuna, 1993). For example, a particular person with epilepsy may only have seizures during sleep or in the early morning, therefore limiting, but not eliminating, a person's driving ability. Even if a student's seizures are not controlled by medication, participation in the classroom portion of driver education should be allowed. Driver education in general has many benefits, such as teaching safety, and is a useful course of study for everyone. When a student's seizures are controlled, the student will be allowed to drive, therefore benefiting from the driver education.

Most states have created guidelines for persons with epilepsy to obtain a driver's license. Usually, medical verification that the person has been seizure free for a particular period of time is needed. For example, in 1994 the states of Alabama, Arkansas, and Mississippi required a one-year seizure-free period; South Carolina, Tennessee, Utah, and Wisconsin established a three-month time period, while Colorado and Connecticut had no set seizure-free period (Driving & Epilepsy, 1993). Based on a model driving law recommended by epilepsy organizations, the state of Nebraska adopted a three-month seizure-free period for drivers with epilepsy (Driver Law, 1994). School personnel should consult the State Department of Motor Vehicles in their particular state for the current regulations pertaining to driving automobiles and students with epilepsy.

Summer Camp

Students planning to go to summer camp may wish to attend a camp with staff that are sensitive to their particular needs. Parents/guardians sometimes ask educators for direction and guidance in locating facilities that are open to students with special needs. An excellent resource for educators who wish to assist parents is *EPILEPSY USA*, a resource newspaper produced by the Epilepsy Foundation of America. Each year a compilation of summer camps that have an interest in serving youngsters with epilepsy is listed. In addition, the organization produces a booklet in this area, titled *The Child With Epilepsy At Camp—A Guide For Counselors.*

Other Activities

Students with epilepsy should be allowed the opportunity to do everything that is presented to other students. Common sense, along with an idea of what the student's abilities are, usually is the guiding rule. Other educators should be made aware of the student's seizures and what procedures to use if one occurs. According to Rowland (1990), "There is no evidence that any particular form of athletics—including contact sports—is more likely than others to precipitate seizures" (p. 252).

When participating in activities that require head protection, all students should be protected by wearing a helmet. Bicycle riding, horseback riding, roller skating, roller blading, skate boarding, and ice skating are among the activities that require head protection.

Summary

There is a tendency for many educators, along with parents, to overprotect the student with epilepsy. Overprotection tends to harm the student and does not allow for participation in typical risk taking of students. Overprotection also implies that the student is being viewed differently from others. We should allow the student to take a risk, thus allowing for the freedom to be like others. Common sense, with an eye for safety, is the guiding rule. "When seizures are well-controlled, most patients [*sic*] can safely ride bicycles (with a helmet), swim, camp, hike, ski, operate machinery, and compete in contact sports so long as they remain in the company of others capable of helping if a seizure occurs" (Dodson et al., 1991, p. 190). We need to remember that "in today's culture, sports and athletic activity are extremely important to young people and that unnecessarily strict interpretation of medical conditions may in fact do more harm than good" (American Academy of Pediatrics, 1983, p. 884).

FROM THE CLASSROOM:

[A school nurse states . . .] "The only problem we've experienced is some overprotectiveness."

Chapter 6

THE STUDENT WITH EPILEPSY AS LEARNER

Some students with epilepsy do very well in school and have few academic problems. Other children have difficulty learning, adjusting, and behaving within the classroom. Some students with epilepsy have other disabilities that influence their learning and adjustment in school. Consequently, there are a number of educational options for students with epilepsy.

One way to look at educational options has been through the various classroom placements based on the individual needs of the person. For example, a student may receive an education through options such as the regular classroom with or without supplementary services, resource room, special class, special school, hospital instruction, home instruction, or residential school. These placements or services have been created to attempt to meet the individual needs of students. One of the prime needs of this population of students is the recognition of the student with epilepsy as a learner. This section will present an overview of numerous facets of learning abilities and disabilities of students with epilepsy.

There are a myriad of factors that affect the student as learner. A word of caution, however, must be given first. If you truly expect to see problems, you are more than likely to find them. Don't look for something that may not exist or is not a problem. Knowledge that a student *could* have a problem allows you to be more sensitive to a particular situation.

There are numerous factors that could interfere with learning. The literature has often noted that significant influences include seizure type, frequency, and cause, as well as medication side effects. These influences can impact a number of areas such as intelligence, attention, memory, behavior, academic underachievement, etc. A range in the degree of problem can exist, such as from small interruptions in attention to permanent impairment in cognition (Binnie, Channon, & Marston, 1990).

INTELLIGENCE

The intelligence range for persons with epilepsy, as measured by standardized IQ tests, is the same as the general population. There have been discussions about some investigations showing a slight, but not significant, reduction in intelligence scores, possibly due to other factors such as medication effects. Students with epilepsy are present in all areas of intelligence. The students can be gifted learners, average achievers, or severely limited.

Svoboda (1979) stated that seizures generally do not affect one's intelligence, unless the seizures occur often and are quite severe. Dodrill (1986) reported that repeated, large numbers of seizures (i.e. tonic-clonic, status epilepticus) could affect intellectual, neuropsychological, as well as the emotional and social abilities of an individual. It appears that the intellectual function in persons with epilepsy is influenced by a number of factors, including age of onset of seizures, duration of the epilepsy, frequency of seizures, types of seizures, cause of seizures, hereditary factors, psychosocial issues, and drug therapy.

ATTENTION

A prerequisite to all learning is being able to pay attention to the task. Schools require students to attend for various amounts of time. There are many reasons why a student may not pay attention in school. Lack of interest, poor teaching, and meaningless curriculum could be influences. Medication, brain injury, and lack of a fully developed nervous system could also be contributing factors.

MEMORY

One of the commonly reported cognitive deficits in individuals with epilepsy has been memory difficulties. Svoboda (1979) noted the existence of poor memory recall, problem-solving abilities, and disorganized work approaches. Memory, however, can be influenced by a number of factors, such as the type of seizure, duration, origin, frequency, and medications. With status epilepticus, there have been some discussions concerning the loss of knowledge of academic skills, resulting in the need to relearn information. There is no strong evidence that status epilepticus impairs long-term memory. However, it is known that the longer the seizure activity, there is an increase in chance of injury to the brain.

Different parts of the brain have different associations. For example, the left temporal lobe is often associated with verbal memory, while the right temporal lobe is related to nonverbal memory. It is the area of the brain affected and the type of seizure that determine the kinds of memory problems that a person may experience. Individuals with simple and complex partial seizures have more memory problems than individuals with generalized seizures. Along the same line of thought, a study by Jambaque, Dellatolas, Dulac, and Signoret (1992) examined children 7 to 14 years of age with partial epilepsy (temporal lobe) and found that they scored lower on all memory tasks compared to the control group.

There are also time factors associated with memory and seizures. For example, it has often been mentioned that there could be an impairment of functioning just before the actual seizure activity. Some individuals may even forget what they were doing just before the seizure. The same principle applies immediately after a seizure, as noted by Dodson et al. (1991) when they stated, "First, it is the experience of most neurologists and primary care physicians that after a first seizure, patients remain somewhat confused and do poorly on standard memory tests even after they appear—at least outwardly—to have recovered from the acute effects of the seizure" (p. 168). In addition, early onset of seizures tends to put a child more at risk for cognitive dysfunction, regardless of the type of seizure (O'Leary, Lovell, & Sackellares, 1983).

Drug therapy can affect many aspects of a person's cognition and memory. Vining (1987) found that phenobarbital affects short-term memory, concentration, and symbol manipulation, while phenytoin interferes with attention, problem solving, and visual motor abilities.

In one study, individuals with epilepsy who were over the age of 15 and were without cerebral lesions were found to have significant memory impairments (Loiseau, Strube, & Broustet, 1983). No reason such as type of epilepsy, frequency of seizures, duration of the condition, or type of medications being taken could fully account in a clear manner for the impairment.

BEHAVIOR PROBLEMS

Students with epilepsy exhibit more behavior problems than other children. They also have more behavior problems compared to other children with chronic diseases. Svoboda (1979) stated that learning problems and behavior disorders are both present in about half of all individuals with epilepsy, and there is a similar number of children experiencing difficulty adjusting to school.

There have been recent investigations concerning the effects of drugs on behavior. In one study parents saw the children who were on valproate behaving inappropriately, while the opposite was true when the children were taking phenobarbital (Vining, Mellits, & Dorsen, 1987). For additional information, see the chapter on medications.

While noting that psychosocial problems are common in students with epilepsy, Henriksen (1990) commented that some children get caught in a vicious cycle "with seizures leading to learning difficulties, and then to school problems, psychosocial problems, and more seizures" (p. s23). The author noted that "the label 'epilepsy' may have a masking effect, causing both the patient and the teacher to blame all of the child's problems on the epilepsy" (p. s24).

SELF-CONCEPT

Students with epilepsy have a more impaired self-concept when compared to students who do not have epilepsy. Hauser and Herdsdorffer (1990) attributed social isolation and stigma as contributing factors. Dodrill (1982) noted the problems of social stigma and discrimination associated with seizures when he stated that "the intermittent appearance of the disorder tends to keep the people around the patient, as well as the patient him or herself, on edge" (p. 112). (See Chapter 7 for further information on this topic.)

ACADEMIC UNDERACHIEVEMENT

There are numbers of studies concerned with academic underachievement of students with epilepsy. The findings from the studies show mixed results.

While past research has found a relationship between academic achievement in arithmetic and seizure type and frequency, Mitchell, Chavez, Lee, and Guzman (1991) did not. In fact, the authors noted "most important, there appears to be no relationship between severity or duration of seizure disorder or total exposure to anticonvulsant drugs and underachievement" (p. 71). It was noted that if a relationship exists between epilepsy and underachievement, it may have more to do with the neurologic abnormalities than with the seizures themselves. This statement is in line with Svoboda (1979) who felt that learning problems in this population originated not so much from the epilepsy but more from the brain itself.

The relationship of age of onset of epilepsy, type of epilepsy syndrome, seizure type, and seizure frequency and school achievement was investigated (Huberty, Austin, Risinger, & McNelis, 1992b). The results indicated that there were no significant relationships between the variables and scores on achievement tests. There was also no relationship between the variables and student retention and no relationship between retention and type of seizure. However, students with generalized seizures were likely to be retained in a grade.

In another study it was found that students with epilepsy made less academic progress than expected, taking into consideration age and IQ (Seidenberg et al., 1986). It was found that the greatest difficulties were first in arithmetic, then in spelling, reading, reading comprehension, and word recognition. In particular, children with generalized seizures performed more poorly in arithmetic than those children with partial seizures. Children with both types of generalized (absence and tonic-clonic) seizures did more poorly than children with any other seizure type. In addition, the authors noted that individuals with more than one type of seizure disorder were often more at risk for problems.

A survey of parents with children with seizure disorders was conducted by the California State Council On Developmental Disabilities (1992). One of the results was that "about two thirds of the children have experienced difficulties keeping up in school, and 44% report a lot of difficulties keeping up in school" (p. 72).

ACADEMIC DISABILITIES

The academic achievement of students with epilepsy is behind other students of the same age (Farwell, Dodrill, & Batzel, 1985). The researchers found more errors on language tasks and, in addition, stated that intelligence correlated with the amount of seizure control.

Freeman et al. (1990) noted that there is a higher incidence of dyslexic type learning problems in students with epilepsy. It was stated that in addition to this concern "another type of learning problem might be associated with problems in hearing, attending, word recognition, and the association of words with memories" (p. 241). Svoboda (1979) noted that children who have an early onset of epilepsy were more likely to have learning problems.

Hauser and Hersdorffer (1990) stated that "academic difficulties, unrelated to characteristics of the epilepsy, may exist among children with epilepsy" (p. 346). They noted the difficulties may include problems in reading accuracy and reading comprehension, behavior, verbal abilities, attention, spelling, arithmetic, language, and memory. While children with epilepsy scored lower on achievement tests as compared to other students, "older children with epilepsy did worse than younger children on tests of spelling, reading comprehension, and arithmetic" (Hauser & Herdsdorffer, 1990). Overall, nearly one of every four children with seizures may need some type of special educational service (Svoboda, 1979).

There is a question, however, as to whether the interference with the learning is due to the epilepsy or some other factor, such as medication side effects. Due to a selection bias in many of the studies, the question concerning the effect of epilepsy on learning needs to continue.

LEARNING ABILITIES/COGNITION

Individuals who have seizures often have cognitive difficulties (Loring & Meader, 1993). There are a number of factors that can contribute to this interference in cognition. For example, Loring and Meader (1993) stated that "age at onset, seizure type and frequency, etiology, cerebral structures affected, psychosocial stressors and antiepileptic medication" (p. 1) can be determinants of the effect. Prolonged and frequent seizures are often related to more severe effects on cognition (Dam, 1990).

Huberty, Austin, Risinger, and McNelis (1992a) found that children with secondary generalized epilepsy did not do as well on test measures as children with other epilepsy syndromes. The findings suggested that a seizure disorder related to brain injury that is associated with generalized seizures is more apt to be a factor in learning problems than generalized, idiopathic seizures.

Dam (1990) found that children with epilepsy have poorer concentration, lower mental processing, and are less alert than an age-matched control group. There were differing degrees of impairment resulting from epilepsy, ranging from mild to severe. The author noted, however, that prolonged and repeated seizures were more related to effects on cognition.

Cognitive performance and educational achievement were investigated in students who were learning disabled. The study involved this population of students with and without epilepsy. The results indicated that students with learning disabilities and epilepsy do not have specific types of learning impairments compared to students with learning disabilities who do not have epilepsy (Vermeulen, Kortstee, Alpherts, & Aldenkamp, 1994).

Consideration must be given to the characteristics of the students used in the investigations. There are other disorders that may, indeed, affect a particular sample of students' learning. For example, Huberty, Austin, Risinger, and McNelis (1992a) noted that the children with epilepsy and mental retardation were not included in their study. It is important to remember that knowing that a student has epilepsy does not tell us anything specific about the educational needs of that particular student (Dreisbach et al., 1982). The relationship between cognition and epilepsy is quite complex.

The use of drug therapy has an affect on the cognition of some students with epilepsy. Noting that children with epilepsy have numbers of learning and behavior problems, Trimble (1990) stated that from the current data it appears that phenobarbital affects cognition, with some effects being quite subtle. In fact, the upper levels of the therapeutic range of phenobarbital may be toxic with regard to learning abilities (Rodin, Schmaltz, & Twitty, 1986). Phenytoin also affects cognition in children, and the data noted, according to Trimble (1990), that higher doses of valproate affects performance on psychomotor tasks, but there are fewer cognitive impairments with this drug. Carbamazepine effects vary with the cognitive test being used, but it seems to have less effect on cognition and there is evidence that it seems to improve speed of performance (Trimble, 1990). According to this author, the evidence on the effect of ethosuximide on cognition is mixed.

Phenytoin, carbazepine, and valproate may affect motor functioning (i.e. coordinated hand movements), and phenytoin may be harmful to performing higher cognitive tasks, according to the work of Duncan, Shorvon, and Trimble (1990). On neuropsychological tests, performance was better by children on valproate compared to children who were taking phenobarbital (Vining, Mellits & Dorsen, 1987).

With focal seizures, the part of the brain with the seizure activity may be associated with learning deficits (Svoboda, 1979). For example, the frontal lobe area of the brain with abnormal discharge may affect independent work. According to Svoboda (1979), the left temporal lobe area with abnormal discharge can affect verbal skills and reasoning as well as having the person experience problems with remembering what is heard (i.e., names, addresses, rhymes, etc.). The person may also experience trouble with reading and spelling, particularly if a phonetic approach is used. Difficulty in mathematics may also exist, such as being confused with what to do for the different operations (addition, subtraction, etc.). With seizure activity in the right temporal lobe area, the student may experience difficulty with work that is visual. For example, the student may have a problem recognizing shapes, forms, familiar words, letters, and numbers. Visual motor problems may exist, with writing difficulties, letter reversals, and visual perception problems present. Other perceptual problems may also be seen, such as not knowing left from right and being clumsy (Svoboda, 1979). With abnormal discharge in the bilateral temporal lobe area of the brain, a person may experience processing deficits, memory problems, attention difficulties, and distractability (Svoboda, 1979).

Aldenkamp, Alpherts, Dekker, and Overweg (1990) discussed types of learning disabilities in children with epilepsy: memory impairments, attention problems leading to underachievement, ability to process information, and problem-solving deficits, resulting in cognitive processing disorders. The authors noted that "epilepsy may have a general impact on learning, regardless of its specific features, and thus account for the observation that a disproportionate number of children with epilepsy exhibit learning problems" (p. s13).

RESOURCE:

Division For Physical And Health Disabilities
The Council For Exceptional Children
1920 Association Drive
Reston, VA 22091-1589

Membership is open to individuals who belong to the Council For Exceptional Children and are interested in the education of students with physical and health disabilities. The organization produces a newsletter and a journal, as well as promoting quality education for this population of students.

RESOURCE:

School Alert
Epilepsy Foundation Of America

A program about epilepsy for school personnel. Call your local affiliate of E.F.A. for details or call 1(800)EFA-1000

RESOURCE:

Coelho Jobs Center

Information about vocational counseling, job clubs, placement services and job training can be obtained. More information can be obtained from the Epilepsy Foundation Of America

RESOURCE:

TAPS

Training Applicants For Placement Success. An E.F.A. employment program for persons with epilepsy to obtain job skills, placement, and retention. Call: (800)EFA-1000

EPILEPSY AND OTHER DISABILITIES

Epilepsy, as a disorder itself, is considered to be a major developmental disorder (Hauser & Hesdorffer, 1990). By occurring at higher rates, epilepsy is related to other specific disabilities. Although there are numbers of other conditions related to epilepsy, primary concern here is given to attention deficit disorder, autism, cerebral palsy, emotional or behavior disorders, learning disabilities, mental retardation, multiple disabilities, multiple sclerosis, traumatic brain injury, and tuberous sclerosis due to the close relationship that exists between each of these conditions and seizure disorders.

Attention Deficit Hyperactivity Disorder

A condition that has been the center of many controversies is attention deficit hyperactivity disorder (ADHD). The literature has discussed this condition with and without hyperactivity, the latter being referred to as attention deficit disorder (ADD). The students in both groups have difficulty concentrating for any period of time. The major difference between the two groups of students is the evidence of hyperactive behavior, although many aspects of what has been written about the condition have been questioned (Reid, Maag, & Vasa, 1993). Students with this disorder do not receive special education services unless they also have another disability. The condition is often associated with learning disabilities (Hardman et al., 1993) but is sometimes related to the characteristics of other disorders.

Freeman, Vining, and Pillas (1990) suggested that ADD may be more common in students with epilepsy. While medications may be used to help a student attend to tasks in school, educators should observe the student for any changes in school performance. Communication with medical personnel and parents/guardians may lead to medication and/or dosage changes if needed. Such changes in behavior can often be noted by educators, as they are often the first ones to notice the differences in behavior.

In addition, the Epilepsy Foundation of America (1987) noted that seizure activity within the brain that has not been identified may also affect the student's attention. Gaddes (1985) referred to the child with "subclinical epilepsy" (p. 398) as one who has a condition that is not strong enough to produce seizures but is disruptive to the degree to create chronic hyperactivity. This child would be referred to a neurologist for a medication program that may include anticonvulsive and/or stimulant drugs.

Autism

A definition of autism was presented in recent regulations:

> Autism means a developmental disability significantly affecting verbal and non-verbal communication and social interaction, generally evident before age three, that adversely affects educational performance. Characteristics of autism include—irregularities and impairments in communication, engagement in repetitive activities and stereotyped movements, resistance to environmental change or change in daily routines, and unusual responses to sensory experiences (Department of Education, 1991, p. 41271).

Individuals with autism are not alike. Generalizations about this population should not be made. A good deal about autism remains unknown, recognizing the need for additional research (Hardman et al., 1993).

Hauser and Hesdorffer (1990) noted that seizures occur in 11 to 35 percent of children designated as autistic, noting that in general "the prevalence of epilepsy is more than 28 times that expected in the general population" (p. 344). About one-third of individuals with autism develop seizures as adults, with complex partial seizures being a common type of epilepsy seen in this population (Gillberg, 1991). Seizure disorders in individuals with autism were more common in persons with lower IQs (Volkmar & Nelson, 1990).

Gillberg (1991) stated that "various environmental factors, such as loud noises, stress, chaotic situations, and sleep deprivation, can contribute to the production of seizures in autism" (p. 74). The author stressed the need for a calm yet well-structured atmosphere for this population of students, especially when attempting to reduce seizure activity.

Cerebral Palsy

Cerebral palsy is a disability created from damage to the brain before or during birth. Gearheart et al. (1993) noted that "cerebral palsy (CP) may also be described as a group of conditions characterized by motor disorders due to abnormalities of brain function" (p. 314). Hallahan and Kauffman (1991) stated that "cerebral palsy can, for practical purposes, be considered part of a syndrome that includes motor dysfunction, seizures, or behavior disorders due to brain damage" (p. 347).

Seizures are frequently observed in students with cerebral palsy. According to the research of Hauser and Hesdorffer (1990), seizures occur in about thirty percent of children with cerebral palsy. In reviewing the results of other studies, the authors concluded that the highest prevalence of epilepsy is with the type of cerebral palsy termed hemiplegia and the lowest prevalence was with children with dyskinesia.

Emotional and Behavior Disorders

Emotional or behavior disorders refers to:

- Behavior that goes to an extreme—behavior that is not just slightly different from the unusual;
- A problem that is chronic—one that does not quickly disappear;
- Behavior that is unacceptable because of social or cultural expectations (Hallahan & Kauffman, 1994, p. 208)

Shea and Bauer (1994) identified behavior disorders as "those whose behavior varies in frequency, intensity, and duration from their general education peers to such an extent that it comes to the attention of authority figures, usually teachers, and results in their being labeled as behaviorally disordered" (p. 151).

Children with epilepsy do have more emotional and behavior problems than children without epilepsy (Hoar, 1984).

Depression is also more common in individuals with epilepsy. This may be more related to the stigma effects, medication, or problems with life in general.

Suicide has also been found to be more common in select populations of individuals with epilepsy. Hauser and Herdsdorffer (1990) stated that the degree of impairment, number and type of seizures are factors related to depression in individuals with epilepsy. Individuals with epilepsy are more likely to be treated for psychiatric disorders, but "when population-based samples of individuals with epilepsy are examined, the prevalence of psychosis may equal that in the general population" (Hauser & Herdsdorffer, 1990, p. 253).

Epilepsy, especially temporal lobe epilepsy, has been associated with aggression in the past. However, current studies do not document any relationship.

Learning Disabilities

Learning disabilities as a field of study has created a great deal of controversy, especially with having a standard definition of the disability. The definition of learning disabilities presently accepted and used in IDEA of 1990 (P.L.-476) is the following:

> "Specific learning disability" means a disorder in one or more of the basic psychological processes involved in understanding or in using language, spoken or written, which may manifest itself in an imperfect ability to listen, think, speak, read, write, spell, or to do mathematical calculations. The term includes such conditions as perceptual handicaps, brain injury, minimal brain dysfunction, dyslexia, and developmental aphasia. The term does not include children who have learning problems which are primarily the result of visual, hearing, or motor handicaps, of mental retardation, of emotional disturbance, or of environmental, cultural, or economic disadvantage. (Section 5[b][4])

There are other proposed definitions of learning disabilities, as well. In reality, this population of students has been defined by exclusion. The students are not learning, and they are not classified as being individuals with emotional disturbance, mental retardation, etc. They do not learn in relation to the school's expectations and they are in need of some type of special assistance. The impact of learning disabilities can vary in degree from mild to very severe.

The literature in special education has stated that there are lists of characteristics describing students labeled as learning disabled. It is important to remember that a student with learning disabilities will have some, not all, of the characteristics. This group of students is truly a heterogeneous population. Frequently cited characteristics include hyperactivity, perceptual and coordination problems, academic learning problems, attention and concentration problems, memory and thinking process disorders, social-emotional problems, lack of strategies for problem solving, and various degrees of impulsivity.

The need for individuals concerned with seizure disorders to be knowledgeable about learning disabilities has been stressed in the literature (Jenkins & Brown, 1992). These authors recommended an integrated approach where epilepsy and learning difficulties are assessed at the same time. In this process, assessment is viewed within the context of medical, psychological, and social areas.

Many students with epilepsy show very few or no learning problems. However, some students may exhibit school problems in a variety of ways. The severity, location, and duration of seizure activity, as well as the type of medication, may be related to the performance of certain types of tasks. For example, seizure activity and/or medication effects have often interfered with verbal and language skills, memory, reasoning ability, reading, spelling, writing, perceptual motor abilities, attention and concentration. Learning disabilities in students with epilepsy may be associated with a number of areas, such as memory, attention, and reduced speed of information processing.

Svoboda (1979) stated that a person with a focal seizure disorder that originated prior to six years of age is a candidate for a learning disability. The Epilepsy Foundation of America (1987) noted that there may be seizure activity within the brain that interferes with its ability to handle information, resulting in academic problems involving memory. Being careful not to make generalizations about students, it must be remembered that there are many factors that enter or can interfere with the learning process. Seizures or epilepsy do not cause learning disabilities. The condition is probably more related to the brain dysfunction that causes the seizures than the seizures themselves.

In examining the research and literature in this area, it is unclear as to the relationship between students with epilepsy having normal intelligence and learning problems. Among individuals with epilepsy and no mental retardation, Batshaw and Perret (1986) felt that a higher than usual incidence of learning disabilities existed. However, there are many factors not taken into account by researchers. For example, Hauser and Herdorffer (1990) noted that medication effects, school attendance, selection bias and small sample numbers were examples of factors not fully considered in past investigations. Researchers were often aware of which subjects had epilepsy and which did not (Hauser & Herdorffer, 1990).

Stedman, Van Heyningen, and Lindsay (1982) established the high incidence of failure in schools by children with epilepsy. In particular, reading, arithmetic, and spelling were affected. It was suggested that teachers' underexpectations resulted from not identifying this population of students and not accurately obtaining a true picture of the students' intelligence.

Huberty, Austin, Risinger, and McNelis (1992b) investigated the age of epilepsy onset, seizure syndrome, seizure type and frequency, as well as the adaptive skills of the children with epilepsy. The authors noted the relationship of seizures to students' academic work has been quite inconsistent. Students with epilepsy *may* have certain problems in particular areas of learning. However, Hauser and Herdorffer (1990) are quick to point out that these problems noted in various studies are in areas "which may or may not manifest themselves in a classroom situation" (p. 344). These authors concluded a discussion of learning difficulties among children with epilepsy by stating that "Thus, academic difficulties, unrelated to characteristics of the epilepsy, may exist among children with epilepsy" (p. 314). It also appears that students with learning disabilities and with epilepsy do not have other educational needs compared to students with learning disabilities only.

Mental Retardation

The American Association on Mental Retardation (Grossman, 1983) defined mental retardation as "significantly subaverage general intellectual functioning resulting in or associated with concurrent impairments in adaptive behavior and manifested during the developmental period" (p. 11). In reviewing the literature concerned with epilepsy and mental retardation, Hauser and Hesdorffer (1990) noted that seizures occur in about 8.8 to 32 percent of children with mental retardation. "In approximately half the cases of childhood-onset epilepsy with an identified cause for their epilepsy, the underlying condition is mental retardation or cerebral palsy" (Hauser, 1994, p. s4).

In examining a population of children with epilepsy, Sillanpaa (1992) found a neurological deficit in 39.9 percent of the group, with the most frequent impairments being mental retardation (31.4%), speech disorders (27.5%), and specific learning disorders (23.1%). Strafstrom (1993) stated that epilepsy is quite common in individuals with Down's syndrome trisomy 21. The author noted that all types of seizures can occur in these persons, although tonic-clonic is the most frequent type.

Marcus (1993) investigated the control of epilepsy in 90 children with mental retardation and epilepsy. The author concluded that the control of epilepsy was not related to the level of mental retardation. Abnormal neurological and EEG results also did not affect the quality of the management of the seizure disorders.

Singh and Towle (1993) found that, in their clinical experience, many individuals with mental retardation and epilepsy may be taking more medication than is necessary. Their research findings suggest that the majority of this population often can be treated with a single drug. Poindexter, Bergland, and Kolstoe (1993) also noted the benefits of reducing the concurrent use of more than two antiepileptic drugs and barbiturates with persons with mental retardation and epilepsy. Coulter (1993) points out that the drug treatment selected for an individual with mental retardation will follow the same guidelines as for other people without mental retardation.

In a discussion of individuals with mental retardation, mental illness, and a seizure disorder, Pary (1993) noted the occasional difficulty for persons with mental retardation to be entered into a psychiatric hospital for treatment of a mental illness. The author concluded that there should be no need to add an additional stigma to these individuals when a seizure disorder also exists. Pary (1993) stated that the persons with the three disorders did not do significantly worse on inpatient units within psychiatric hospitals.

Litzinger, Duvall, and Little (1993) had success in integrating individuals with profound mental retardation and epilepsy from an institution to a community group home. Credit was given to the use of new antiepileptic drugs (valproate and carbamazepine), early intervention when dealing with the seizures, and appropriate residential staff education.

Multiple Disabilities

Brimer (1990) discussed multiple disabilities when stating that persons with severe disabilities or multiple disabilities have a very significant functional discrepancy in: "(1) general developmental abilities, (2) caring and looking after themselves, (3) expressing thoughts, ideas, and feelings, (4) responding to environmental stimuli, and (5) interacting socially with chronological-age peers" (p. 110).

There are numbers of disorders that when combined can be included in this definition. However, the focus of this section is with disabilities and epilepsy. When a disability and epilepsy are combined, a special condition exists. Brimer (1990) noted that "It is widely believed that two disabling conditions have an additive relationship (one adds to the other). But in actuality they have an exponential relationship (the effects of one are multiplied by the effects of the other), so that the two are significantly greater in effect than either would be in isolation" (p. 111).

After reviewing the research and literature concerned with disabilities and seizures, Hauser and Hesdorffer (1990) concluded that seizures occur in about fifty percent of children who have both mental retardation and cerebral palsy. Sunder and Davis (1992) examined a population with multihandicaps and found that 29 percent of the group had no seizures, 17 percent had seizures and received no anticonvulsant therapy, 59 percent experienced tonic-clonic seizures, 12 percent had Lennox-Gastaut syndrome and, with the use of medications, 12 percent of the group maintained control and 41 percent of the group had seizures that were uncontrolled.

The California State Council on Developmental Disabilities (1993) reported that over 47 percent of the individuals in their survey stated that in addition to epilepsy they also had some type of health problem, such as asthma or diabetes. Fifty-three percent of the parents of children with seizure disorders reported that their child had some type of health problem.

Multiple Sclerosis

Multiple sclerosis is a neurological condition that involves "the progressive destruction of myelin, the fatty material that covers the nerves of the body" (Wagman, 1983, p. 475). It is characterized by speech problems, muscle incoordination and weakness, and vision problems.

The prevalence of epilepsy (particularly partial seizures) is significantly higher in persons with multiple sclerosis as compared to the general population (Kinnunen & Wilkstom, 1986). The authors stated that there was no correlation between the severity of multiple sclerosis and the acquisition of epilepsy. Noting that seizures might be a beginning symptom of multiple sclerosis in some people, the authors observed that the seizures appeared before any other multiple sclerosis symptoms.

Traumatic Brain Injury

Traumatic brain injury (TBI) is a recognized category of disability under recent federal regulations. It has become a more frequent cause of neurological impairment and is receiving more public and professional recognition. Savage (1988) noted that the National Head Injury Foundation, Inc. defined TBI as

> an insult to the brain, not of a degenerative or congenital nature but caused by an external force, that may produce a diminished or altered state of consciousness, which results in impairment of cognitive abilities or physical functioning. It can also result in the disturbance of behavioral or emotional functioning. These impairments may be either temporary or permanent and cause partial or total functional disability or psychosocial maladjustment. (p. 2)

A definite relationship between head trauma and epilepsy exists, especially for penetrating head trauma (Hauser & Herdorffer, 1990). It is, however, only one of the many consequences of head injury. The Epilepsy Foundation of America (1992a, 1992c) noted, though, that head injury is a significant cause of seizures, which may occur immediately or years after the head injury. It is sometimes recognized as a cause of epilepsy that can be lowered by reducing the number and severity of head injuries. Hauser and Herdorffer (1990) stated that "removing head trauma as a cause of unprovoked seizures or epilepsy would reduce the incidence of epilepsy by only 2–4%" (p. 130). There is, however, an increased risk of seizures after brain injury from the head trauma, particularly in relation to the severity of the injury. It has been estimated that 5 to 10 percent of individuals with traumatic brain injury also have epilepsy (Giles & Clark-Wilson, 1993).

Tuberous Sclerosis

Tuberous sclerosis is a genetic condition concerned with skin disorders, tumors, mental retardation, and seizures. The tumors can be found on the face and throughout the body, including the brain (Carter, 1975). Individuals with tuberous sclerosis can have other deficits associated with having tumors, such as health problems, organ dysfunctions, and mental deterioration (Beirne-Smith, Patton, Ittenbach 1994).

CONCLUSION

The neurological system consists of the brain, the spinal cord, and the nerves within the body. When there is damage to a part of the neurological system, there is often a corresponding effect to another part of the system. Educators must be knowledgeable about these effects upon their students and continue to create valid educational programs that meet each student's individual needs.

A significant number of students with epilepsy do not perform in school at the level expected (Hartlage & Green, 1972; Svoboda, 1979). The problems in school may be due to a number of factors. Svoboda (1979) hypothesized that these problems are probably due to a combination of factors. There is a belief by some educators that students taking anticonvulsant medications have a disability, leading some individuals to have lower expectations of these students (Hartlage & Green, 1972). Others have believed that the associated disabilities present the problem more than the actual seizures (Dreisbach et al, 1982). Another thought is that the problem is a failure by educators to identify students with epilepsy (Stedman et al., 1982).

Students with epilepsy can be gifted, average, or slow learners. They may do well in school or do very poorly. Epilepsy can affect the learning abilities, behavior or achievement of some students. Recognition of the student's individual needs is one of the responsibilities of the educator.

Chapter 7

SELF-ESTEEM, ACCEPTANCE, AND UNDERSTANDING

SELF-ESTEEM

While self-concept is the way one views oneself, self-esteem is a judgment of one's own worth. Students often put their self-esteem on a level based on other people's reactions to them. A student who receives negative reactions from others, such as peers and teachers, will often be prone to negative or lowered self-esteem.

Students with low self-esteem view life in a negative fashion. They feel powerless, often being afraid of taking risks. There is frequently a perception of not having any control over their lives.

There is a great deal of control over the life of the student with epilepsy by parents, educators, and medical personnel. Even in schools, a high degree of overprotection of these students was found (Diaz, Alegria, & Ferrando, 1986). With numbers of restrictions, the student also can develop a degree of dependency. Baroff (1991) noted that a portion of self-esteem that might be affected by these restrictions is the dimension of autonomy. Indeed, a certain amount of freedom, including the opportunity to experience a degree of risk, is needed by all students, including those with epilepsy.

Self-esteem is an important component of the student's overall development. It has a relationship with other critical areas, such as sound social-emotional development, school achievement, and mental health (Pope, McHale, & Craighead, 1988). It is important for the educator to employ strategies that can help all students learn skills that improve self-esteem levels.

A practical model for creating activities to develop self-esteem can be seen in the writings of Garbe (1990) who was concerned with students who were shy. It was suggested to lead students from activities that first require work as individuals, later in partners, then in small groups, and, at a later point, in large groups. A move from little interaction with others to more interaction is the recommended course of action. The author noted that "awareness, understanding, and appropriate teaching strategies helps to create the special mixture it takes to . . . water the shrinking violet" (p. 510).

A very difficult aspect of having epilepsy is not the disorder itself but the problems associated with it (Epilepsy Foundation of America, 1991). Students with epilepsy have a great deal of difficulty in trying to feel good about themselves, even though it is possible to achieve high levels of acceptance for this population (Strixrud, 1988). Epilepsy affects self-esteem as stigma is attached to this disorder (Baroff, 1991). Important to acceptance of epilepsy is self-esteem (Freeman et al., 1990), even though the various threats to self-esteem can be seen in the literature on epilepsy (Baroff, 1991). In fact, Devinsky (1994) stated that "the parents and teachers of children with epilepsy may see them as 'doing remarkably well,' but deep inside, the children may remain insecure and have low self-esteem" (p. 205).

How does a person's perception of self change after a seizure? According to Freeman, Vining, and Pillas (1990), it depends a great deal on the self-image of the individual before the seizure. "The change, if any, will depend on the type of seizure and its immediate effects on him [*sic*], on his developmental age, and on what, if anything, follows the seizure" (p. 215).

FROM THE CLASSROOM:

[A young adult speaks . . .] "I've always been a loner. That's the way it is and has been. In school I stayed by myself—no big deal. Today, I'm still basically a loner. I live by myself and do things by myself. My boss and other people at work know I have epilepsy. I just stay to myself. That's the way I like it."

[An elementary school student speaks . . .] "Sometimes I feel different. I really don't like being different. I want to be like everybody else."

[A young adult speaks . . .] "No one knows [about having epilepsy]. I just tell some people. Otherwise, no one has any idea at all. I just as soon not have them know."

[After having a seizure, a middle school student speaks . . .] "I just want everyone to know

that I'm okay. I want my friends to know that everything's all right."

Educators can play a significant role in developing self-esteem in students. They are the most important persons affecting self-esteem when children begin school. The suggested activities and teaching suggestions are built on a premise derived from the research and literature in this area. It suggests that the following factors are important for all activities and strategies:

- a sense of being important to self and others;
- a feeling of being capable of learning and achieving;
- a development of pride and accomplishment;
- a sense of responsibility to self and others;
- an awareness of having friends; and
- a sense of control over events in school.

Educators are in an ideal position to enhance the self-esteem of students. The following section is composed of activities and teaching ideas. Although this listing is extensive, it is suggested that the educator pick, choose, and adapt any ideas for use with students. In addition, this series is only a beginning to spark the educator's imagination for developing ideas to enhance students' self-esteem.

Daily Journal

A daily or weekly journal of feelings and reactions to events and experiences could be used. The student could write both positive and negative aspects of the day or week. If the journal is not kept private (which could be an option for some students), the educator could use the expressed ideas as a springboard for discussions or for writing back to the student. Dialogue concerning epilepsy could be one area.

Rap Sessions

Group talk sessions help students understand each other and how they are seen by others. The educator can also help students to understand appropriate ways of interacting with others.

Q-Sort

Kroth (1973) has suggested using the Q-sort technique to assist students in analyzing behaviors that could be changed. Students sort descriptive adjectives into piles labeled as "existing" behavior and "ideal" behavior. A goal for change is then established from examining the behaviors within the piles.

Assertiveness Training

Assertiveness is characterized as being honest, direct, sharing, and open. Students feel better about themselves due to their appropriate expressions made about them and others. It is used in social situations and is related to the locus of control concept. Assertive students control situations, while nonassertive individuals allow others to control behaviors, actions and/or situations.

Guess Who?

Have each student in the class write something positive about the student on his/her right. The activity then requires that each student try to guess who the statements are about.

- Match a peer with the student to act as a classroom buddy;
- Have the students make a "success" book, consisting of all the great things that have happened at home and/or school;
- Have the student develop a hobby; encourage this through investigating their interests;
- Assist the student at the beginning of each piece of work in order to ensure a successful start;
- Assign classroom duties; give the student a task that can be completed with success;
- Call attention to success by any of the students;
- Have the student act as a leader of a particular group function;
- Have the student present or demonstrate a skill, activity, hobby, etc., to the class;
- Reduce competition among students;
- Incorporate various cooperative learning strategies into the classroom;
- Have the student tutor or help another student in the class or school;
- Have the student do an independent project or book report on a famous person with epilepsy;
- Make adjustments to the class in order to reduce stress, failure, rejection, etc.;

- Teach the student acceptable ways to deal with rejection, unhappiness, etc.;
- Seat away from others who are not receptive or empathetic to this individual;
- Encourage students to interact appropriately with the student with epilepsy;
- Help the student identify behaviors which may be annoying to others; develop strategies with the student to change those behaviors;
- Explain to the student the difference between making friends naturally and pushing oneself onto others;
- Include fun activities for all students as part of the curriculum;
- Be genuine in your interactions with the student; be sure that situations for involvement are not contrived;
- Help all students improve their physical appearances;
- Take the time to listen to all students' expressed concerns and needs;
- Encourage the student to get involved with appropriate physical activities, such as walking, jogging, tennis, swimming, etc.;
- Give the student with epilepsy, as well as other students, a responsibility on school grounds, such as lowering flags, making announcements, washing blackboards, etc;
- Have the student verbally repeat to the teacher the successes of the day/week;
- Have all students create a "who am I" notebook, consisting of pictures, stories, and drawings about themselves;
- Have students develop relationships through pen pals;
- Evaluate the difficulty of the material the student is expected to learn; aim for a very high correct success rate to increase self-esteem;
- Have the student do one step of the directions or tasks at a time to be sure each step is completed successfully;
- Make sure verbal directions are at a level the student can understand;
- Do the beginning problems or tasks with the student to make certain success is met; work with the student until independence with success is obtained;
- Allow the student additional time, space, materials, assistance, etc. (if necessary) to complete the task successfully;
- Make the topic of self-esteem a center of discussion with the class (Pope, et. al, 1988);
- Allow the student the option of doing a task at some other time of

the day or taking it home, particularly if the student is not feeling well, is tired from seizure activity, or is experiencing medication effects;

- Break longer tasks into shorter assignments with increased success;
- Allow the student to complete certain tasks in a private setting (carrel, study area, corner of room, etc.) to bypass fear of a failure in front of peers.
- Allow the student to "showcase" skills in a variety of ways, such as displaying work on the bulletin board, etc.;
- Share with the parents positive progress being made in the classroom;
- Have parents give praise to the student for success;
- Assign the job of teacher assistant for a specified period of time;
- Match a student with a peer that has similar interests and abilities;
- Allow the student to feel free to communicate with other significant school personnel, such as the school nurse, school psychologist, guidance counselor, etc.;
- Design situations for the student to develop appropriate social skills;
- Keep realistic expectations of the student in mind with respect to the student's abilities and disabilities;
- Allow alternative assignments in order to ensure student success;
- Reward student for success with lunch together with a special staff member, or have a special table and setting for lunch with a classmate;
- Write short personal notes of acknowledgment and encouragement;
- If a task is quite complex, break it down into simpler subtasks that can be completed with success; activities are created that are "do-able" for that particular student;
- Have students collect items that tell about themselves; magazine pictures, objects, and drawn pictures can be used; the students then share with others why and how the items are about them;
- Set easily achievable classroom goals for the student;
- Record progress of the student; share growth with student and family; progress toward the goal can be pointed out to the student frequently;
- Conduct class sessions where questions about epilepsy, health, safety, etc., can be posed, answered, and discussed;
- Students often reflect their environment; if their surroundings reflect interest, warmth, love, and desire for learning, students will often

act accordingly; if the classroom is disorganized and in disrepair, the students will not take pride in their classroom and in their work. Pride, responsibility, and organization are quickly reflected in classrooms to students;

- Foster sensitivity for other students, as well as respect for oneself and other students (Pope et al., 1988);
- Focus on positive strengths of the student;
- Encourage the student to make friends who will be accepting;
- Be an active advocate for the student;
- Involve the parents in building self-esteem;
- Show unconditional support for the student; be there for the student in crisis situations and afterwards;
- Communicate with the student in a personal, sincere manner; often students perceive that no one understands what they are going through. In addition, nonverbal communication sends a message to the student with epilepsy. Facial expressions, eye contact, confidence in first-aid procedures, and acceptance of the student are quickly recognized.

COMMERCIAL PROGRAMS

In addition to teaching strategies, commercial programs may be useful since they often deal with a number of different issues which may be useful in developing various aspects of a student's self-esteem. For example, personal identity, human relationships, awareness of feelings, communication, social skills, problem solving, and examining individual strengths and limitations play an important role. There are many companies that produce materials to assist in increasing all students' self-esteem. In addition, commercial programs may be useful in helping students learn to accept individual differences, as well as acquire a level of disability awareness. The following companies have produced materials in this area:

Academic Therapy Publications
20 Commercial Boulevard
Novato, CA 94949-6191

American Guidance Service
4201 Woodland Road
P.O. Box 99
Circle Pines, MN 55014-1796

Developmental Learning Materials
7440 Natchez Ave.
Niles, IL 60648

Eye Gate Media
Jamaica, NY 11435

Hawthorne Educational Services
800 Gray Oak Drive
Columbia, MO 65201

Human Policy Press
P.O. Box 127
Syracuse, NY 13210

Listen and Learn Company
3366 Pescadoro Rd.
LaHonda, CA 94020

Research Press
P.O. Box 9177
Champaign, IL 61826

The Kids Come In Special Flavors Co.
P.O. Box 562
Dayton, OH

RESOURCE:

College-bound students with epilepsy can obtain valuable scholarship information through:

Parke-Davis Epilepsy Scholarship Program
c/o IntraMed
1180 Avenue of the Americas
New York, NY 10036
Phone: (800) 292-7373

The educator is the key to sound self-esteem development in the schools. The affective growth of the student is as important as the academic side. How educators act and react to and with students affects students' views of themselves (Hayes & Fors, 1990). Hopefully, the school in conjunction with the family will foster every child's growth in this area.

The importance of self-esteem cannot be overemphasized. To have students build their self-esteem in realistic ways, educators must realize that a particular time slot in the school day devoted to increasing "self-esteem" is not sufficient. How the educator treats students, reactions and attitudes toward seizure behaviors, and helping students feel good about themselves are areas that the educator must focus upon throughout the entire school day. In fact, "the teacher-student relationship and the school environment may play a more significant role than direct instruction" (Hayes & Fors, 1990, p. 211). Respect, honesty, and trust must be incorporated into the school environment.

ACCEPTANCE AND UNDERSTANDING

Educators have the responsibility of helping others understand and accept the student with epilepsy. As Cartwright, Cartwright, and Ward (1984) stated, "Perhaps the greatest hurdle for children with convulsive disorders is the social and emotional trauma of rejection by peers and adults who are uninformed and unsympathetic about the disability" (p. 144).

Acceptance and understanding within the schools can be approached from several ways. The first is through the student, having safety and care for the person being a priority. The student must have an understanding of epilepsy and the particular seizure disorder to the extent appropriate. Expectations of the student within the classroom should be consistent with other students of similar ability. Secondly, other students within the classroom and school must be familiar with the disorder and safety procedures to be followed. The presence of the student in the school can give the educators the opportunity to present realistic lessons dealing with helping others, first aid, compassion, etc. Epilepsy education in the classroom helps students understand the disorder and may help others develop an appropriate attitude to individuals with epilepsy (Austin & Fraser, 1993). Another factor is the school personnel's reaction to seizures. The way one handles a crisis is often reflected to others.

FROM THE CLASSROOM:

> [**A school nurse states...**] **"We developed information packets on various disorders for use by everyone in the school. Only the essential information was included, as well as what to do in an emergency situation. One of the disorders included in the package was epilepsy."**

DEALING WITH STUDENT'S FEELINGS

The educator can help significantly by acknowledging the student's feelings about seizures. This is particularly important if we wish to deal realistically with acceptance and understanding. Some suggestions for the educator, other school personnel, and peers within the classroom include:

- Utilize individual listening time; give the student uninterrupted, individual time to listen to what has to be said; try to avoid interruptions, give no comments, and present no interpretations. Just listen!

- Show compassion and understanding; reflect back to the student what was said; restate in your own words what was said by the student; it is often the unpredictability of the seizure that leads to feelings of helplessness, fear and loss of control.
- Be reassuring and supportive; acknowledge the feelings that the student expresses; don't lecture or attempt to negate what the person feels; allow the student to express, to vent, and to channel feelings into words.
- Allow alternative means of expression to occur; for example, allow the student to draw pictures of the feelings being experienced or have the student express feelings through journal writing.
- Don't put the student down when feelings are being expressed; keep away from making the incident trivial, as it may be most important to the student; encourage the student to verbalize, giving the tools of important coping skills.
- Discuss the meaning of "feeling" words such as embarrassed, lonely, guilty, confused, etc.; make a list of these words, discuss them, and use and apply the words in different situations.
- Be aware of your own feelings toward the student's seizures; your attitude and behavior can easily be detected by the student and others in the classroom and school; it is often people's reactions to a seizure that create concerns.
- Suggest counseling by the school psychologist; this strategy may help the student understand and gain a degree of self-control; this type of goal could be obtained through counselor strategies such as learning progressive relaxation, self-instructions, and memory aids (Frank, 1985).

TEACHING OTHER STUDENTS ABOUT EPILEPSY

To build acceptance and understanding, other students in the school must have a knowledge about seizures and epilepsy. The other students should have an understanding of what goes on during different types of seizures (Potolicchio, 1992). If there is a student with epilepsy in your class, obtain parental permission prior to beginning teaching other students about the condition. You may also want to have the student with epilepsy involved in planning and implementation of the lessons. They may want to know, in advance, what aspects of the condition are going to be taught. With this advance notice, it also allows the parents the opportunity to express any concerns they may have. However, if the student or parents wish anonymity, those wishes must be granted. A direct and honest approach should be used.

- Show understanding and knowledge, not fear; with young children, stress that seizures are not painful and not contagious; with older students, the educator can discuss causes and treatment of seizures;
- Answer all questions honestly;
- Use group counseling sessions conducted by the school psychologist; Frank (1985) suggested that this strategy be used with students who may have witnessed a seizure; "the psychologist can present information about epilepsy at a level the children can understand, answer their questions, explore their fears, and suggest positive ways for them to interact with the epileptic [*sic*] child" (Frank, 1985, p. 201);
- Explore other students' feelings and concerns about epilepsy and seizures;
- Discuss how other students can help during a seizure;
- Have other students take an active role in dealing with this disorder; for example, sending letters when any student is out of school for a period of time is often practiced or having students assist with first-aid procedures gives an important and active role to play during this crisis;
- Stress the important facts about epilepsy to the students during the class discussions; maintain the level of discussion appropriate to the students' ability to understand; don't tell the students more about epilepsy than they are ready to know; Points to include in the discussion to help students understand could include:
  (1) What was seen is called a seizure (or epilepsy);
  (2) No one will be hurt or will die; sometimes it just looks scary;
  (3) When the brain gets a lot of different messages, the body acts this way (the degree and amount of information will depend on the needs of the particular group of students);
  (4) A seizure (or epilepsy) is not a disease and you can't catch it;

(5) When the seizure is over, everything returns back to the way it was; it is only a temporary problem (or some people say inconvenience);
(6) Discuss with the class that head injury can cause epilepsy; emphasize safety with discussions about the use of helmets, speed reduction in cars, and the use of seat belts;
(7) Have students role play first-aid procedures to be used for the different types of seizures;
(8) Note the things that people do that they normally don't do during a seizure; "treat reactions to loss of bladder control in a matter-of-fact manner" (Oliver, 1983, p. 25). Emphasize empathy.

- Discuss the different feelings of the person who experienced the seizure;
- Generate ways the class can help the person feel good about him/herself;
- Invite a person with epilepsy to be a guest speaker in your classroom; your local affiliate of the Epilepsy Foundation of America may be able to assist you;
- Have the students in your class write reports on famous people who had epilepsy (i.e., U.S. Representative Tony Coelho, Bobby Jones of the Philadelphia 76ers basketball team, etc.); and
- Videotapes of seizures and first-aid procedures could be shown (Potolicchio, 1992).

Oliver (1983) suggested teaching about epilepsy within the context of the health curriculum. A number of issues that can be applied to everyone can be used, such as "personal concerns about competence, confidence, and control of self as well as life planning and vocational or career concerns. As part of the health curriculum, epilepsy is an example of one among many disorders which can affect a person's life style" (p. 4).

FROM THE CLASSROOM:

[A teacher states . . .] "We explained to the class [third grade] that just like telephone wires can sometimes cross and the signals get mixed up, the messages along our nerves sometimes cross and that our muscles get those mixed messages and contract and relax too fast. This is what might have happened to their friend in the classroom.

"We have to have education of students so that children with seizures are not treated as oddities or outcasts."

RESOURCE:

"Count Me In!"

A collaborative project between the Epilepsy Foundation of America and the National Association of School Nurses; resources for the school nurse include videotapes, comic books, manuals and other materials dealing with epilepsy.
Contact the Epilepsy Foundation of America: (800) EFA-1000

USING BOOKS AND STORIES

Reading books and stories can be used to help individual students and classmates understand epilepsy and seizures. Discussions about the book can lead to increased knowledge and empathy. Books about children with epilepsy can help develop a positive view of individuals with the disorder. Students can learn to respect the differences that exist among people. As Slapin, Lessing, and Belkind (1987) stated: "The wonderful thing about books is that they are plentiful, relatively inexpensive, and can be strong forces in attitude formation and role modeling. Stories can be read, reread, memorized, changed, adapted, and used as a starting point for a variety of classroom activities, such as art, drama, songs, and craft projects. Books open doors to ideas" (p. 2).

It is important to avoid books and stories that depict individuals with epilepsy in a stereotypical manner. Stories that have messages that are incorrect, misleading, or handicapist must be avoided. Thought must be given to the selection of books that are age appropriate, applicable to the situation, are attractive and motivating, and do not contain stereotypes.

Examples of literature that educators may find useful include:

Lee the Rabbit with Epilepsy by Deborah M. Moss. Rockville, MD: Woodbine House, 1989.

This illustrated book was written for children ages three to six years old. The story is about a rabbit who has seizures, visits a doctor, and receives treatment. The book can be used as a springboard to explain epilepsy and the treatment to very young children.

Dotty the Dalmatian has Epilepsy by Dr. Wellbook. Tim Peters & Company, 1993.

This 16-page book was written for children between the ages of two and six. The reader finds that Dotty the dalmatian has epilepsy and is afraid and embarrassed. But Dotty learns to accept and control the seizures and goes back to helping the fire fighters.

My Friend Emily by S.W. Swanson. Writers Press, Boise, Idaho, 1994.

This small book is appropriate for young children. It is especially useful for teaching other students in the classroom about the disorder.

A Child's Guide To Seizure Disorders by the Epilepsy Foundation of America, 1987.

This small pamphlet is but one example of the materials that can be obtained from the Epilepsy Foundation. Elementary school children will find this pamphlet useful, particularly when an adult assists the child in filling in the blanks (i.e., my seizure is called ______, my medicine is ______).

Me and My World—All About Epilepsy by the Epilepsy Foundation of America, 1981.

This 45-page book can be used with elementary school age and beginning middle school age students. The book tells the reader about epilepsy, seizure types, medications, other students reactions, and how epilepsy affects people.

Seizure Man, First Aid For Seizures by the Epilepsy Foundation of America, 1990.

This eight-page comic book explains appropriate first-aid procedures for seizures. The book is recommended for use with children five to eight years of age.

Because You Are My Friend by the Epilepsy Foundation of America, 1982.

A young boy discusses epilepsy, seizures, and what first-aid procedures should be used. An important aspect of the 16-page pamphlet is the discussion of why his friend's understanding is important and needed.

I Have Epilepsy by A. Braithwaite. London: HarperCollins, 1993.

Appropriate for elementary students, the book explains epilepsy from a young person's viewpoint. This is a very readable book for students who want to learn more about the condition. However, individuals may find the author's use of the word "fit" offensive.

Mike Has Epilepsy by Geigy Pharmaceuticals, Ardley, NY, 1983.

This small booklet discusses epilepsy and is appropriate for students in the elementary school.

Dreams Come True by Katie Kornfield
Rocky Mountain Children's Press, Boise, Idaho 83712

The story is about having epilepsy, appropriate for students between the ages of six and ten. Using pictures from the family album, the photo/story booklet is written in Katie's own words.

Julia, Mungo, & The Earthquake by Saxby Pridmore and Mary McGrath, Magination Press, NY, 1991.

This story about epilepsy was written for students between the ages of three and ten. The story is about a young girl with epilepsy who overcomes barriers typically faced by others with epilepsy.

Mom I Have A Staring Problem by Marion and Tiffany Buckel (P.O. Box 20833, Bradenton, FL 34203-0833), 1992.

Written from the view of a seven-year-old, the small book describes the various experiences encountered by the young girl with absence seizures. It is a true account of how the child's seizures were related to a learning disability. This book could be used with upper elementary school age and middle school students.

Trick Or Treat Or Trouble by Barbara Aiello and Jeffrey Shulman, Twenty-First Century Books, From "The Kids on the Block" series, Columbia, MD.

This book was written for children between the ages of eight and twelve. Learning that epilepsy is not to be feared, students read an adventure tale.

Spider-Man Battles the Myth Monster by the Epilepsy Foundation of America.

This 16-page comic book presents the lives of three children who have either epilepsy, asthma, or diabetes. Excellent reading for students between the ages of nine and thirteen for promoting understanding of health conditions.

A Season of Secrets by Alison Cragin Herzig and Jane Lawrence Mali, Little, Brown and Company, Boston, 1982.

This 193-page book is appropriate for middle school students. The mysterious fainting spells, which were not explained by the parents, are of concern to the older sister. Epilepsy and seizures are explained within the context of the story.

A Handful of Stars by Barbara Girion, Charles Scribner's Sons, New York, 1981.

This 179-page book is appropriate reading for middle and high school students. The story presents the trials and tribulations of a teenager whose life changes due to her epilepsy.

Answers to Your Questions About Epilepsy by the Epilepsy Foundation of America, 1982.

Factual information that is beneficial for teenagers is presented. The 32-page booklet uses examples to answer questions about epilepsy and marriage, jobs, driving, drinking, and drugs.

Alice by Sara Flanagan. St. Martins Press, 1988.

This 306-page book is appropriate for teenagers. The story is about a young girl with epilepsy and a hearing impairment. With the help of two new friends, she begins to learn. The story was the basis of the television movie *Wildflower.*

Epilepsy by Tom McGowan, Franklin Watts, 1989.

This 94-page hardcover book is very useful for high school age students. The book discusses various aspects of epilepsy as well as the history of the condition.

Seized by Eve LaPlante, Harper Collins, 1993.

This 254-page hardcover book could be used by high school students and adults to learn about a particular syndrome associated with temporal lobe epilepsy. The author presents current, relevant information about this disorder, and then illustrates the effects of this syndrome by presenting the lives of three individuals who have the disorder.

Brainstorms: Epilepsy in Our Words by Steven C. Schachter, Raven Press, 1993.

This 197-page book might be useful for some high school students or young adults. Due to the detailed, sensitive, personal descriptions of seizures, the educator should preview this book carefully before recommending it to a specific student. The reader can also learn how epilepsy affects people.

The Brainstorms Companion—Epilepsy In Our View by Steven C. Schachter, Raven Press, 1995.

This book contains descriptions of seizures in the words of friends, family members, and acquaintances of individuals with seizure disorders. Similar in nature to the preceding book, the content is quite sensitive and the educator must use judgment prior to recommending it to a high school student.

RESOURCE:

Books Without Bias
A Guide to Evaluating Children's Literature For Handicapism by Beverly Slapin, Jill Lessing, and Elaine Belkind.

A guide to help you ask the right questions about books and stories that have characters with disabilities

RESOURCE:

"Kids on the Block" Book Series
The Kids on the Block, Inc.
9385-c Gerwig Lane
Columbia, MD 21046
Phone: (410) 290-9095
Toll Free: (800) 368-kids

Books written for children between the ages of 8 and 12. The books, authored by Barbara Aiello and Jeffrey Shulman, teach children about individual differences.

Secrets Aren't (Always) For Keeps Learning Disability
Trick Or Treat Or Trouble Epilepsy
It's Your Turn At Bat Cerebral Palsy
Business Is Looking Up Visual Impairment
Friends For Life AIDS

Hometown Hero Asthma
A Portrait Of Me Diabetes
On With The Show Divorce

RESOURCE:

KID'S NEWS

Epilepsy Foundation of America

As a free insert in *Epilepsy U.S.A.*, this is a publication that spotlights children with epilepsy. The newsletter contains artwork, letters, pictures, and information about epilepsy for young children. It also presents an opportunity for students to share ideas with others.

Chapter 8

MEDICATION AND RECORD KEEPING

MEDICATION OVERVIEW

Typical treatment for epilepsy is the use of medications called anticonvulsant or antiepileptic drugs. Many educators come in contact with students on such medications (Gadow, 1982). These medications do not cure epilepsy but only prevent, or reduce the number of, seizures. About seventy percent of persons on medication will have seizures controlled, while another 20 percent will have seizures occasionally. The remainder will have seizures that will impair their functioning.

Medications can be used singularly or in combinations. Although there are numbers of medications that can be used, the following are typically seen:

Trade Name	Generic Name
Clonopin	Clonazepam
Depakene	Valproic acid
Depakote	Divalproex sodium
Dilantin	Phenytoin
Felbatol	Felbamate
Gabapentin	Neurontin
Klonopin	Clonazepam
Lamictal	Lamotrigine
Luminal	Phenobarbital
Mysoline	Primidone
Tegretol	Carbamazepine
Tranxene	Clorazepate
Zarontin	Ethosuximide

The choice of drugs for the treatment of epilepsy is made based on the type of seizure, along with a number of other factors. Medical personnel can select from several types of drugs for each type of seizure. Numbers of different kinds of medications are available and new drugs are being developed in order to treat this condition. The goal is to control the seizures with the fewest number of drugs (Baroff, 1991).

Individuals react differently to the various drugs and doctors can customize the dosage and/or the choice of drug. The way to choose the most appropriate medication is to have a physician correctly identify the type of seizure, which then directs the doctor into appropriate drug selections (Dodson et al., 1991). It was found that physicians, nurses, and adults with seizures rated medication information as a most important learning need about epilepsy (Dilorio, Faherty, & Manteuffel, 1993).

Medications can have side effects, even when the student is receiving the correct dosage. Students react differently to medications, some experiencing side effects while others do not. Depending on the drug used, side effects from anticonvulsive medications typically include:

- drowsiness
- sleep disturbances
- hypoactivity
- memory deficits
- nausea
- skin rashes
- cognitive impairment
- aggressiveness
- weight gain
- hair loss
- blurred vision
- incoordination
- problems with sensory discrimination
- hardening of the features of the face
- irritability
- distractible
- fussiness
- fatigue
- lethargy
- hyperactivity
- lack of attention span
- dulled thinking abilities
- dryness of mouth
- vomiting
- excitability
- depression
- increased appetite
- nystagmus
- dizziness
- gingervival hyperplasia (gaps created between the teeth and the gums)
- lowered self-esteem
- fine motor function problems
- emotional swings
- clumsiness
- hirsutism (excessive hair growth on the arms, face, legs, etc.)

Svoboda (1979) stated that there are four types of drug reactions. The first type is intoxication, as seen when a person has taken too much of a drug. The second type is an allergic reaction to the medication by the body. The third type is an idiosyncrasy of an unexpected drug reaction, while the last type is a malformation created by a drug taken during pregnancy that creates an effect on the fetus. The educator should pay particular attention to the first three types of reactions and report any occurrences that may be observed. For example, the student may not be as alert as usual, reaction times may be slowed down, or be very drowsy. The student may be observed as being clumsy, even to the point of appearing to be in a drunken state. Falling asleep easily, the student cannot focus on the work. Svoboda (1979) noted that the heavily intoxicated child may stagger in a stupor, fall easily, vomit, and the breathing may be slow and shallow. At the other end of the spectrum, educators should keep in mind that it could take a period of time (possibly up to two weeks) for the medication to be at the appropriate level to be effective (Forness & Kavale, 1988).

Reactions to specific medications can also be seen. For example, Gadow (1979) noted that phenobarbital can produce drowsiness, irritability, and hyperactivity; mesantoin's effects include drowsiness; mysoline creates double vision, dizziness, and ataxia; and zarontin can produce nausea, vomiting, loss of appetite, abdominal pain, and hiccups. Gillberg (1991) stated that valproic acid sometimes bring "anorexia, vomiting, and aggression" (p. 73), and carbamazepine has some children who have seizures and autism "become more repetitious and stereotyped" (p. 73).

Additional concerns about phenobarbital have been expressed, such as increased irritability and sleep disturbance (Camfield et al., 1979), interference with sustained attention (Hutt, Jackson, Belsham, & Higgins, 1968), and decreases in intellectual development (Smith & Wallace, 1982). However, other studies, such as Wolf et al. (1981), have not shown the effect of this drug on cognitive functions. The effects of drugs, however, can be best be viewed in a general sense: "Polytherapy and high levels of any antiepileptic drug are likely to cause cognitive and behavioral side effects" (Santilli et al., 1991, p. 67). (See Chapter 6 for additional information on this topic.)

Bergen (1991) stated that "the aim is always to use them [antiepileptic drugs] in doses adequate to control seizures but low enough to avoid unwanted effects" (p. 18). But it was noted that "almost all AEDs have been found to have unfavorable effects on attention, learning, motor skills, and intellectual performance" (Bergen, 1991, p. 18). These effects, though, can range on a continuum from very small to profound. It has been suspected that it is possible that all antiepileptic drugs could affect neurological functioning to some degree.

FROM THE CLASSROOM:

> [A special education teacher states . . .] **"When you mention medication, I immediately think of the side effects, especially on behavior. Some of them [students] are fast asleep and others are climbing the walls."**
>
> [A school nurse states . . .] **"We have had many children with seizures, both grand mal and petit mal. Most of the petit mal were breakthrough seizures, indicating a need for a change or increase in medication.**
>
> **"The student felt strange. He had a known history of seizures. The nurse was called by the teacher and the administrator was notified and he responded as well. The student was assisted to the floor for safety by the nurse, reassured verbally, and supported during the seizure. The parent was notified, the ambulance summoned, and the student was transported to the local hospital with the parent for evaluation and treatment. A private physician had changed the medication and the school was not advised."**

Many anticonvulsant medications can be administered at home before and after school. When medications cannot be given at home, the school nurse should be contacted. ***The educator must be familiar with the school district's policies regarding the administration and handling of medication.*** Many school districts do not allow students to carry any medications, requiring the parent/guardian to bring the medication to the school nurse's office in the original container.

Information is needed by the educator in order to effectively work with a student on medication. The parents/guardians should obtain critical information which might be useful to school personnel. For example, some guiding questions to achieve this goal would include:

- What medication is the student to take?
- What are the typical side effects of the medication?
- How does the medication help the student?

- What changes in behavior might be seen?
- How often and for how long does the student have to take the medication?
- When does the student take the medication?
- What are the indicators that may be seen regarding the intake of either a toxic or inadequate dosage of medication?

The use of antiepileptic drugs is the medical approach to the treatment of students with epilepsy. Individualized programs that address the learning and behavior problems of students are also necessary. Dreisbach et al. (1982) "recognized that effective management of children with epilepsy requires more than treatment with anticonvulsant medications" (p. 119). More recently it was stated that

> our findings suggest that attention simply to seizure control in the clinical setting will not address the full range of problems of children with epilepsy. These results also indicate that the need for programs that prevent development of psychological, social, and school performance problems of children of children with epilepsy. (Austin, Smith, Risinger, & McNelis, 1994, p. 613)

RECORD KEEPING

The recent laws and regulations have recognized the rights of students with epilepsy and acknowledged the importance of educators understanding the needs of this population. With this recognition of rights, there is a demand for accurate educator observation of seizures (Epilepsy Foundation of America, 1987). Educators are in an ideal position to identify behaviors which may lead to the medical diagnosis of epilepsy. Accurate observations are also needed to provide physicians with objective information which could be used for seizure control and classification, choice of medications, etc. This information may also alert physicians to events (i.e. time of day, medication, flashing lights) that might precipitate seizures.

Recognition of an undetected seizure disorder within the classroom has a special importance to the members of the Epilepsy Foundation of America. The Silver Owl Award, or other types of recognition, is given to teachers who first recognize that a student has a seizure disorder. The certificates, usually presented by Epilepsy Foundation affiliates, honor the educator and bring public awareness of the disorder. Additional information about the award can be found in the last chapter of the book. According to a newspaper article from the Epilepsy Foundation of

America (Silver Owls, 1990), "Recognition of an undetected seizure disorder in a child is not only an important step in understanding and treating the condition, it also prevents learning disabilities caused by forced periods of inattention" (p. 4). Trippi (1989) discussed the need for physicians, parents, and service providers to monitor the effects of medication on individuals. Although the responsibility for the administration of medication is with the parents/guardians and physician, the educator plays a vital role in the observation, recording, and reporting of behavioral changes which may originate from the medication side effects. Trippi (1989) recommends the use of a drug therapy information sheet which would be completed by the physician. Examples of the information included on this form are the contact person in case of an emergency, medication dosage, behaviors to be observed, cautions and possible side effects, and care implications. Educators, having use of such information, would benefit in the monitoring of drug effects on their students. Before beginning any observation system, however, the educator should examine the school district policy regarding medications.

FROM THE CLASSROOM:

[A school nurse states . . .] "Parents are asked to supply a medical history as well as any other information that may help us to aid the student, such as any signs of an oncoming seizure, physical, emotional, etc."

"Some parents don't tell that the child could have a seizure until one occurs in school."

"We had a student have a grand mal seizure in the hall between classes. The parents had never informed the school that he had a history of seizures and was on daily medication. An ambulance was called before we could reach the parent. It was most embarrassing for everyone concerned."

"Students with an undisclosed seizure disorder are at risk on the stairs, in gym class, climbing ropes, or even in the swimming pool."

[A school nurse states . . .] "We must have parents keep the school informed and up to date on daily limits, restrictions, medications, etc."

Michael (1992) described a simple procedure, using a Seizure Observation Form, to document objective information concerning seizures in the classroom. In addition, the author presented guidelines, consisting of a number of questions, to assist the educator in observing seizure activity. The use of such procedures and guidelines may be useful in the medical treatment and educational interventions planned for the student.

Based on the work of Zeigler and Erba (1983) and appropriate record keeping systems suggested by the Epilepsy Foundation of America (1981), the Seizure Observation Form and the Guidelines for Seizure Observation are presented in Figure 3 and Figure 4, respectively.

To use the Seizure Observation Form (Figure 3), the educator views

Student's Name—John

Date of Seizure—3/13/90
Time of Seizure—9:00 am
Approximate Duration of Seizure—2 minutes

Behavior Before Seizure—John appeared to be tired and complained of a headache. He was resting at his desk, putting his head down on his arms.

Initial Seizure Behavior—He let out a short cry. His whole body appeared to stiffen.

Behavior During Seizure—John fell to the floor. His whole body, including his arms and legs, began to jerk violently. His eyes rolled upward and his eyelids were fluttering. John had lost consciousness and fallen to the floor. His facial skin was very pale and his lips were bluish. The seizure lasted about two minutes.

Behavior After Seizure—John was very tired and wanted to rest. He complained that he had a severe headache.

Student Reaction to Seizure—John was quite upset and confused. He didn't seem to understand what had happened.

Peer Reaction to Seizure—At the time of the seizure, other children were not in the room. However, the children in the room should be made aware of the seizure, given an understanding of the behavior, and taught basic safety procedures. It was recommended that I call the local epilepsy foundation and the national Epilepsy Foundation of America (4351 Garden City Dr., Landover, MD 20785) for additional assistance.

Teacher Comments—John was not injured. The school nurse assisted with the incident and the parents were notified. John's fears and concerns need to be addressed. I will begin by obtaining help from the local epilepsy foundation. The parents, school nurse, and guidance counselor will assist me in helping John address his concerns.

Figure 3. Seizure Observation Form. SOURCE: Michael R. J. (1992). Seizures: Teacher observations and record keeping. *Intervention in School and Clinic, 27*(4):212. Reproduced by permission.

the student's behavior before, during, and after the seizure. The date, time, and approximate duration of the seizure are important aspects to be recorded. The student, peer, and educator reactions can be used for subsequent educational interventions.

The Guidelines for Seizure Observation (Figure 4) consist of a series of questions that act as a guide for observing seizures with more precision. It can also help the educator in obtaining a more complete and thorough observation. This can be accomplished by reflecting on the guideline questions prior to observing a seizure in the classroom. With increased awareness, educators can be alert to events that might precipitate seizures (Patton, Payne, & Beirne-Smith, 1990).

In order to assist the educator in gaining insights about the information needed in the Seizure Observation Form, there are questions posed in the Guidelines for Seizure Observation Form. Figure 4 (Michael, 1992, p. 212) is presented as an example of the information that may be taken from observing a seizure objectively.

When a seizure occurs in school, parents/guardians are to be notified, as per the school district's established procedures. There are some students, however, who have such frequent seizures that reporting each one to the parents becomes inappropriate. In these instances, "a weekly report or summary of seizure activity may be more appropriate" (Bergen, 1991, p. 18).

To augment verbal descriptions of the classroom behaviors associated with seizures, the use of videotape might be considered. After obtaining permission to videotape the occurrences in the classroom, the educator can present concrete examples of the observed behaviors to the parents and/or medical personnel. While Gibbs and Appleton (1992) used family home videos to document and demonstrate the child's seizures, a comparable technique could be used by educators in the classroom. School administrator, parent/guardian, and medical approvals should first be obtained.

SAFEGUARDING RECORDS

Information about a student with epilepsy can be collected and used, but it must be dealt with care and with appropriate safeguards. Educators have the responsibility to safeguard educational records.

To protect students and families with respect to information collected, safeguards were originated in the Family Education Rights and Privacy

Before Seizure Activity	During Seizure Activity	After Seizure Activity
What was the child doing prior to the seizure?	What was the level of consciousness during the seizure?	Did the child have:
Did the child appear to be ill or feverish?	Was the child's body rigid or limp?	A sense of drowsiness or confusion?
Was the child recently napping?	Were there any sudden jerking movements of the body or arms?	Any difficulty in regaining consciousness?
Did the child sense anything different? sensations smells extreme fatigue drowsiness excitement headaches verbalizations facial skin coloration staring excessive anxiety hyperventilation	Did the child appear to be sweaty, flush, or pale?	Any weakness specific to one side of the body, arms or legs?
	What were the child's eyes doing? (i.e. rolled upward, turned to the left or right, eyelids fluttering, etc.?	Any problems with vision?
	Were there any episodes of automatisms, (e.g. lip smacking, picking at clothes, fumbling, wandering around room, etc.)?	Any recent changes in child's medication (i.e., dosage, type, etc.)?
	Was there any evidence of twitching? Where did it begin? Did it progress to other parts of the body?	Was any injury sustained?
	Was there any occurrence of vomiting or incontinence?	
	Was there any evidence of cyanosis?	

Figure 4. Guidelines for Seizure Observation. SOURCE: Michael, R. J. (1992). Seizures: Teacher observations and record keeping. *Intervention in School and Clinic, 27*(4):213. Reproduced by permission.

Act of 1974, which provides minimum requirements for maintaining records (Valente, 1980), and the Education for All Handicapped Children's Act of 1975. The family and student have a right to privacy, and informed consent to collect information must be obtained by the schools from the parents. According to Hartshorne and Boomer (1993), "Any form of information collected, maintained, or used by the school that relates to a child is considered an educational record and must be safeguarded" (p. 33). Records, such as medical evaluations, which do not originate from the schools but are put in the student's file are also included within this law (Hartshorne & Boomer, 1993).

Parents and students who are 18 years of age or older have the right to examine the information within a student's file. School officials of the school district or school officials of another school or agency that the student will be going to also can examine records. Parents and eligible students who think that information in the records is inaccurate and/or a violation of student's rights can request that the records be changed. Schools may give information to other education and social service agencies without permission of the parents, but the school must keep a record of these requests. With written parental consent, information from the files may also be given to others such as a physician (Hartshorne & Boomer, 1993).

Information concerning what to keep and what to include in school records was discussed by Cartwright et al. (1984). Originating from a conference by the Russell Sage Foundation, three types of information were noted by the group. Category A was basic information needed by the schools, such as attendance data and report cards. Category B was information that was documented, such as a medical condition. Category C was concerned with information that needed informed consent, such as assessment data.

CONCLUSION

Medications play an important role in the treatment of epilepsy. Medical personnel select the appropriate drug(s) for treatment. Observations of any reactions or side effects is necessary. Educators can play a vital role by observing and recording behaviors in an objective and systematic fashion. Such information can provide physicians with insights that can be used for the control of seizures, the selection of medication(s), and the determination of possible seizure precipitants.

Chapter 9

SAFETY PROCEDURES

Providing a safe environment for all students is a goal for many schools. Basic safety procedures concerning students with seizures are presented here for educators and other school personnel. Everyone who comes into contact with students—administrators, teachers, school nurses, support staff, school crossing guards, etc.—must be given accurate and complete safety information. Individuals should also examine the school policies concerned with medical emergencies. The following procedures are taken, in part, from the Epilepsy Foundation of America (1981, 1989, 1991) and various researchers (i.e., Driefuss, 1988; Jan et al., 1983; *Neurologic Disorders,* 1984) in the field. The procedures are presented for each type of seizure.

TONIC-CLONIC SEIZURE

- Remain calm;
- If the student has not fallen to the floor, help down to a horizontal position;
- Loosen any tight clothing; remove eyeglasses;
- Move any hard or sharp objects, classroom furniture, toys, etc., away from the student;
- Cradle the person's head, if necessary, or put something soft, such as a towel or coat, underneath the head to protect it;
- If possible, turn the person's head to the side to allow accumulated saliva to flow out;
- *Don't* restrain the person or do anything to interfere with the movements;
- *Don't* attempt to stop the seizure;
- *Don't* put anything in the person's mouth; it is impossible to swallow the tongue (Jan et al., 1983);
- *Don't* give any food or drink until the person has fully recovered;

- If the seizure is febrile in nature, keep the body cool by sponging with tepid water;
- There is no need to panic if it appears that the person has stopped breathing for a short period of time; give artificial respiration only if the person does not resume breathing after the seizure ends (Epilepsy Foundation of America, 1992c);
- If the seizure lasts longer than five minutes or a second seizure occurs immediately after the first seizure, have the person taken to a medical facility immediately (Epilepsy Foundation of America, 1991); if the person is pregnant, injured, or diabetic, call immediately for medical assistance (Epilepsy Foundation of America, 1991, p. 6);
- After the seizure ends, let the student rest in the company of an adult;
- Be reassuring, supportive, and comforting when the person gains consciousness; some individuals are embarrassed after the episode;
- Give slow, simple statements to the person, as there are periods of confusion immediately after the seizure; allow sufficient time for the person to process what is being said;
- Reassure the person that the feelings and any mobility problems are temporary (*Neurologic Disorders,* 1984);
- Allow the person to rest; some individuals are extremely tired after seizure activity; after a period of time, encourage activity only to the extent that the person can handle it;
- Tell the student what has happened; in most cases the person has no recollection of the seizure; attention and memory may be affected (Ridgeway & Like, 1991);
- Remember that the student, if safety procedures are followed, will not get hurt and will not hurt others;
- Post-seizure considerations are important; reduce stimuli, such as confusing sounds and noises, and eliminate other sounds such as televisions, telephones, intercoms, excessive talk and opening and closing doors (Ridgeway & Like, 1991).
- Inform the student's parents/guardians, school administrator, school nurse, and appropriate medical personnel, as per one's school policy;
- Do not bring up the subject of seizures and epilepsy as a constant reminder to the student and peers in the classroom; there is more to the student than seizures;

- Continue to treat the student as you would any other students in your classroom.

FROM THE CLASSROOM:

[A school nurse states . . .] "The child was having his first seizure in the classroom. The teacher said she had been taught to put something in the child's mouth to keep him from swallowing his tongue. She put her fingers in his mouth and was bitten. The teacher ended up in the emergency room!

"It can be a frightening sight to students and adults who are unprepared."

[A school nurse states . . .] "The seizure was witnessed by the teacher who became near hysterical. The child was on the floor, dazed, and profoundly exhausted. I calmly explained to the student and teacher what had happened and what was going to be done for her. Unfortunately, she [the student] had to be transferred to the hospital via ambulance.

"Information [about epilepsy] should be a 'natural' component of health training."

[A school nurse states . . .] "I've been involved with school staff training on a one-to-one basis. If a student has a seizure disorder, I explain it to each teacher involved with the student, including what his or her seizure looks like, how long it is likely to last and what they can do to help."

ABSENCE SEIZURE

Students with absence seizures do not require first-aid procedures; however, it is necessary for everyone involved with the student to be aware in order to prevent accidents. For example, a danger could exist if the student was working with a dangerous tool in technology class, was in a high place in physical education class, or was in a location that required balance.

If absence seizures are first suspected, the parents/guardians must be notified in order for them to obtain a medical evaluation of the student's condition.

SIMPLE PARTIAL SEIZURE

The student with simple partial seizures does not require first-aid procedures unless it turns into a convulsion. However, the student needs a great deal of emotional support and reassurance.

COMPLEX PARTIAL SEIZURE

The Epilepsy Foundation of America (1992c) recommends the following procedures be used with individuals experiencing a nonconvulsive complex partial seizure:

- Do not restrain the person;
- Remove harmful objects from the person's path;
- Calmly try to encourage the person to sit down and encourage him or her away from dangerous situations. If the person does not respond to these measures, force should not be used;
- Observe but do not approach the person who appears angry or combative;
- Remain with the person until he or she is fully alert. (p. 12)

In addition, the teacher should speak calmly to the student but remember that you cannot expect instructions to be followed by the student. Also, keep in mind:

- Safety of the student is first; remove any harmful objects;
- Do not grab or shout at the student;
- Steps and windows could be dangerous places; guide the person away;
- Call for assistance only if the student becomes aggressive or dangerous;
- Remember that what is seen is unconscious behavior; any form of punishment or reprimands are quite inappropriate;
- Be reassuring and comforting.

There is a need for educators to have a knowledge about this particular type of seizure disorder (Yard & Thurman, 1982). According to these authors, difficulty in seizure management can be evidenced since many interventions may be started that are based on the assumption that the behaviors are initiated and controlled by the student. Therefore, it is feasible that these seizure behaviors may be misinterpreted as emotional or behavior disorders.

Frank's (1985) opinion is that psychomotor (complex partial) seizures create the most problem in the classroom due to the disruption. "A child experiencing a psychomotor seizure may become belligerent, boastful, or antagonistic and may even have a temper tantrum, roam meaninglessly around the building, or destroy property, again without choosing to do so and without conscious awareness or later memory of what is happening" (p. 201). These seizure behaviors are not under the control of the student, and intervention strategies typically used with students with emotional disabilities/behavior disorders will not be effective.

FROM THE CLASSROOM:

[A school nurse states . . .] "We must maintain student privacy, self-esteem, and dignity while at the same time deal with safety issues."

[A school nurse states . . .] "The biggest problem I've seen is that the student doesn't want to talk about it and usually feels very upset and embarrassed after a seizure."

STUDENT SAFETY AND FIRST-AID SKILLS

Students should be taught safety and first-aid skills, appropriate to their abilities. A qualified individual could be brought into the classroom for such instruction. Often another student is the first person to notice an incidence that requires assistance. Stem and Test (1989) stated that first-aid skills that could be taught include:

(1) Mouth-to-mouth resuscitation;
(2) Water safety;
(3) Fire safety/mild burns;
(4) First aid for poisoning;
(5) Pressure points for bleeding;
(6) Treating falls;
(7) First aid for seizures (p. 11)

According to the authors, the skills *not* to teach because of difficulty to learn and because the use of incorrect procedures could be dangerous to the person include:

(1) CPR;
(2) Lifesaving skills;
(3) Treating severe burns;
(4) Using tourniquets;
(5) Making splints;
(6) Treating eye injuries;
(7) Injury rescue and short-distance transfer. (p. 11)

In an article by Stem and Test (1989), the authors taught students with moderate mental retardation some basic first-aid skills. The teaching was done through teacher modeling of skills, student imitation, and practice, teacher prompting for incorrect procedures, student practice, and the use of mock situations. For example,

> You and your friend are out at McDonald's eating lunch. Your friend is laughing and talking while eating and begins to choke on a piece of hamburger. He first begins to cough. Then he is unable to cough, breathe, or speak. What do you do? (p. 12)

Appropriate scenarios involving seizures could be used to have students prepared to assist a peer having a seizure. With increased knowledge, students can be active participants dealing with safety issues in our schools.

Guynn (1983) discussed the pairing of individuals through a buddy system for the support needed for an individual with a chronic condition. According to the author there were two main purposes for the system:

(1) Facilitate transition of the student to the school and assistance with daily activities; for example, keeping the student with the chronic condition informed about school activities and assignments if the student has been absent from school; and
(2) Use as a helper in emergency and crisis situations in school; an important activity under this purpose would include the buddy attending a half-hour training program at the hospital to learn about the chronic condition and necessary procedures used to give assistance. Awards were presented to each helper.

The author suggested that such a system can be a part of the overall school's comprehensive health plan. In addition, "Having a buddy' to identify with allows the special need student to feel 'less different' in an environment that is alien and intolerant of differences" (Guynn, 1983, p. 625).

FROM THE CLASSROOM:

[A school nurse states . . .] "The teacher panicked and many of the children were crying. All seemed terrified except one child whose mother had seizures at home. This child was kneeling down, gently rubbing the student's hand and he had pushed the adjacent desks away."

[A school nurse states . . .] "Other students bring her to me [the school nurse] when she does not feel well. Her description of this is that 'she feels weird.' She stays with me and I call the mother."

"The other students were ushered to one side of the room. After the seizure was over, the student involved was taken to the health office and later that day a class on seizure disorders was conducted for that particular class. The students handled the situation well."

[A school nurse states . . .] "I think every staff member—teaching as well as support staff and bus drivers—should be trained in the understanding of and immediate response to an incident."

"You have to keep the bus drivers in mind. Kids have had seizures on the bus and the driver has to pull over. He's by himself to deal with the problem."

"Our bus driver on the special education bus has had the experience. She has a child with a seizure disorder. This child has seized on more than one occasion on her way to school. Her monitor is with the children on the bus. In general, though, the bus drivers are nervous about the seizures."

[A school nurse states . . .] "The bus drivers attend a course and refresher sessions. Seizures and the bus drivers are usually addressed in the

course or refresher sessions that are held once a year. I usually add to or explain the film that is shown."

THE SCHOOL ENVIRONMENT AND SAFETY

The physical school environment must be safe for all students. There are, additionally, some basic precautions (including avoidance of seizure triggers) that the school can take into consideration for the safety of students with epilepsy. The ideas are suggested and should not be overplayed, as the goal is to maintain independence as much as possible for this population of students. The environmental factors are presented for consideration by school personnel. This listing is only a beginning and many other ideas could be added, particularly in relation to the needs of a particular student.

- Pad sharp edges of classroom furniture;
- Sharp protruding objects (i.e. faucets, water spouts) should be covered with soft material;
- Purchase school furniture with rounded corners;
- Use carpeting on the floors when possible;
- Cover and/or barricade exposed heating sources;
- Keep clutter out of hallways and passageways in the classroom;
- Use shatterproof materials (mirrors, cookware, etc.);
- Have blankets or other soft materials available to use for protection if needed;
- Use non-skid strips in the gym showers; have grab bars available;
- Limit the use of electric irons, hand-held hair dryers and top of stove cooking with those individuals with frequent seizures with a loss of consciousness (Spitz, 1992);
- Be sure shower drains are working properly; drownings can occur in very shallow water;
- Avoid the occurrence of flashing lights; replace flashing fluorescent classroom lights that are worn; maintain computer monitors;
- Maintain comfortable temperatures within the classroom and the school; avoid excessive cold or hot temperatures;
- Outdoor play activities for all students should be on soft areas (i.e. grass, soft ground, etc.);
- Use helmets for students who need head protection;

- Safety on the school bus must be emphasized, particularly the use of seat belts;
- Depending on the type, frequency, and severity of seizures, students with epilepsy may be told not to use stairs; the use of the elevator with a buddy may be more appropriate; and
- Be sure *all* individuals in the school environment (i.e. cafeteria monitors, school bus drivers, etc.) know first-aid procedures for seizures.

HOSPITALIZATION

Generally speaking, seizures do not require hospitalization of the person. However, there may be times, depending on the needs of the student, when hospitalization must occur. Driefuss (1988) stated that a person should go to a hospital if the seizure lasts longer than ten minutes, the seizures occur one after another, or the seizures are overlapping.

The process of reentry into school for a student with a long absence requires coordinated efforts by health and school personnel, family members, and the student. A plan for successful school reentry by a student with a chronic condition includes the planning and work of the total school health team (Sexton & Madan-Swain, 1993).

FROM THE CLASSROOM:

[A teacher states . . .] "The student was in computer class. It was later determined that the computer screen may have 'triggered' the seizure."

[A school nurse states . . .] "A student was acting strangely and calling out. She was brought to the health office. While we were trying to determine what was happening, she went into a full-blown seizure. We laid her on the floor and protected her from harm. Her seizure lasted approximately four to five minutes. She was not verbally responsive until she was ready to go to the hospital. She had not had any seizures in years. The class had been working with the lights off in the room. They were showing bright colors as part of a science lesson. The doctor felt it was the lights and colors that triggered the seizure."

A student who misses school for periods of time should get extra help or assistance in order to make up the work. Temporary home or hospital instruction may be an option. In some cases, an itinerant teacher may be used to provide instruction to the student and act as a liaison between the student's regular teachers and the student. Some schools have also used closed-circuit television and computer connections through telephone lines to establish ties with the student who may be absent for an extended period of time.

RESOURCE:

Medic Alert Bracelets and Neckchains
Seizure Disorder Identification

Medic Alert
Medic Alert Foundation International
Turlock, CA 95381-1009
Phone: (800) ID–ALERT

Chapter 10

THE FAMILY

OVERVIEW

The competent educator recognizes the importance of working with the student's family. Parents or guardians can, in particular, play an important role in helping the student to reach the educational goals established. The influence of the family on the educational process is being acknowledged by educators. "Professionals should seek out the special insights that parents can offer by virtue of living with their exceptional child" (Hallahan et al., p. 448).

There are several models of the stages or processes that a family may go through when they realize that their child has a disability. Typically, the stages that the family may experience include shock, denial, guilt, anger, sadness, and acceptance. However, there are variations of these stages in different models. For example, the stages of parents with a child with a physical disability may include shock and disruption, denial, sadness, anxiety, anger and fear, and, finally, gradual adaptation leading to reorganization and long-term acceptance (Drotar, Baskiewicz, Irwin, Kennell, & Klaus, 1975). A general model was developed by Gargiulo (1985) that included three major stages: (1) initial shock, followed by denial, grief and depression; (2) ambivalence, followed by guilt, anger, shame, and embarrassment; and (3) bargaining, adaptation, and reorganization leading to acceptance and adjustment.

It is important to note that parents do not go through these stages in a particular sequence, nor do they experience them in any set amount of time. In fact, parents may jump from stage to stage or even skip a particular reaction. Patterns of responses by families are extremely variable, highly individual and personal.

There are many issues and problems confronting the family of a child with epilepsy. The family may face stigma, discrimination, health care costs, problems associated with school absences, and the child's lowered self-esteem. With having a child with a disorder, the family can feel shock, disbelief, disappointment, and stress. In fact, many parents, when witnessing a seizure for the first time, thought that their child was dying or had died (Baumer, David, Valentine, Roberts, & Hughes, 1981). Parents of children with seizure disorders have expressed very high levels of anxiety and depression after it has been determined that their child had epilepsy. Mitchell (1992) identified "parents' vulnerability, search for a reason, fear of injury or death of the child, uncertainty about the next seizure, worries over the child's adult life, and loss of control leading to overprotection" (p. 15) as areas of concern by parents with children with epilepsy. Many families have fears concerning this disorder but, often, it is based from a lack of knowledge about epilepsy (Austin & Fraser, 1993). In addition, the parents may blame each other or try to deny the existence of the disorder.

> **[A mother of an infant states . . .] "I feel tired. My whole family feels the results of having a baby with infantile spasms. We have been going from specialist to specialist—one city to another. It's been hectic. We've been looking for some answers to our questions and we can't find them. I guess we'll just keep looking."**

Children with epilepsy and with behavior problems were found to have poorer seizure control and tended to be in families that were troubled (Austin, Risinger, & Beckett, 1992). In fact, the mothers of the children, according to the same researchers, were getting less support from relatives. "The finding that children experiencing behavior problems tended to be in families that were also experiencing stress suggests that interventions designed to address behavior problems in children with epilepsy should be both family centered and focused on reducing family strain" (Austin et al., 1992, p. 1120).

> **[A mother with a child with uncontrolled seizures states . . .] "What I really need is another person to talk to that is going through the same thing as I am."**

> **[A mother states . . .] "No one should be alone when going through something like this. I find it terrifying. I want my child to be okay. I wonder what will happen in the future."**

The assumption should not be made that having a child with a disorder, such as epilepsy, automatically affects the family in a negative fashion. In fact, it has been reported that, at times, there have been some unexpected positive outcomes within the family of a child with a disability. For example, increased concern for others, acceptance of individual differences, and closer family ties have been reported (Hallahan & Kauffman, 1994).

> **[One father and mother state . . .] "We [the family] are closer now than ever before. We are working on this together. Everything gets discussed and we decide on our every move together."**

In a survey of parents with children with seizure disorders, one of the findings concerned with dissatisfaction with schools noted that the most common response dealt with educators' lack of training and knowledge in dealing with students with seizure disorders, as well as with the related issues associated with this condition (California State Council on Developmental Disabilities, 1992).

Svoboda (1979) noted that "parents all too often leave planning for their epileptic [*sic*] child up to others: they tend to give up, to accept inferior programs, or to allow their feelings to be overlooked. This places a smaller load on the school, but the child suffers" (p. 199). The family, indeed, needs the educator's assistance and support. The educator is truly a part of the team that helps the family cope.

RESOURCE:

The National Parent Network On Disabilities
1600 Prince Street, Suite 115
Alexandria, VA 22314
Phone: (703) 684-6763
Fax: (703) 836-1232

Advocacy for the rights of children with disabilities and their families; membership includes a newsletter, legislative updates, reports, training sessions, and meetings.

COMMUNICATION WITH THE FAMILY

Communication with the family is vital. Determine what the concerns are for their child at school. How can you help them? How can you support their efforts? Sometimes, allowing them to voice their problems and concerns is the first step to take. Opening up lines of communication with the family establishes a firm foundation for your relationship.

An effective way to maintain communication is through the use of a traveling notebook (Hallahan & Kauffman, 1991). It is a notebook of brief messages that goes back and forth among concerned parties. It allows the professionals and parents the opportunity to keep updated as to what is going on with the student. Various individuals can have input into the traveling notebook, such as the teacher, school nurse, parents, neurologist, etc. Lines of communication are kept open on an informal, yet effective and frequent, manner.

FROM THE CLASSROOM:

[A school administrator states . . .] "Our problem has been with the parents. It almost seems that they don't care. How are we going to help the child when the parents don't make sure the medication is taken?"

[An administrator of a private school for students with disabilities states . . .] "We have had a lot of success using the notebook as a way for everyone involved with the child to communicate and to keep in touch with each other. It's quick and it's simple. It's also a nice way for any of the staff to be able to let the parents know what is going on with the child. And it really doesn't have to be of tremendous importance—a short note home on the wonderful accomplishments of the week works wonders!"

WORKING WITH THE FAMILY

One of the recommendations that can be made to parents is getting involved with a parent support or advocacy group. Belonging to such a group is a useful way for parents to learn coping skills, new information, and ways to get needed services. Such a group may serve as a means of obtaining emotional support. They can focus on the problems and issues that are of particular importance to them. Other benefits of parent groups include "(1) alleviating loneliness and isolation, (2) providing information, (3) providing role models, and (4) providing a basis for comparison" (Seligman & Darling, 1989, p. 44). Informal sources of support, such as groups and clubs, are often more effective than formal supports (i.e. professionals) in helping the family adapt and deal with a child with a disability (Kauffman & Hallahan, 1991). Educators can and should help families to help themselves, particularly if one wishes to enhance the quality of life for the student with epilepsy (Coulter & Cerreto, 1993).

The parent and family network of the Epilepsy Foundation of America can help you put a parent/family in contact with another parent/family in order to communicate with and to provide support for each other. Use the EFA toll-free number as a means to obtain this resource for parents/guardians.

RESOURCE:

EPILEPSY FOUNDATION OF AMERICA
Phone: (800) EFA-1000

The importance of family involvement with the student's education cannot be overestimated. In fact, federal and state laws mandate parent participation in various aspects of the student's education. For example, among the rights held by parents of a student with a disability include:

- Issuing written permission before testing for special education services is given;
- Consenting to a change in placement (either in or out) of special education services;
- Participating in the planning of the child's IEP;
- Having another person, such as an advocate, friend, attorney, etc., be present at any facet of the IEP meeting;
- Having their child educated with students without disabilities to the extent that the program is appropriate;
- Knowing what records are kept on their child and having the right to examine and duplicate them;
- Obtaining a full evaluation of the child's present level of functioning; if the parents disagree with the results, an independent evaluation can be obtained. In many situations, the school district is responsible for the costs of this evaluation;
- Having a due process hearing that will obtain an independent review of the child's evaluation or educational program;

- Giving permission for individuals (other than particular school personnel) to view records of the child;
- Knowing their parental rights; schools must keep parents informed of what the school plans are for the child;

> [A mother states . . .] **"We keep records of everything—conversations with key people, medical information, past IEP's, educational evaluations, progress reports, notes from teachers, notes from telephone calls with key people, drug prescriptions, possible side effects of medications, major concerns of the family. It's all there—you name it and I have a record of it. And it's all neatly catalogued in my files at home. You never know when you may need a piece of information quickly. Keep records of everything and keep it organized!"**

RESOURCE:

Information and Guidance
Legal Advocacy Dept.
Epilepsy Foundation Of America
Phone: (301) 459-3700

Working and communicating with the parents/guardians is a significant part of the role of an educator. Establish rapport with the parents and realize that your attitude and feelings toward epilepsy and seizures are quickly conveyed to the parents.

Don't trivialize the parents' concerns for their child. They are real and of importance to them. Use the parents' knowledge about their child and the particular type of epilepsy to learn more about the child and the disorder.

Obtain suggestions from the parents about program improvement. If applicable, discuss their involvement with the IEP meeting as well as the progress made by the student toward the goals and objectives written into the program. Communicate in jargon-free language.

Do not make generalizations about students with epilepsy. They are all different, as other children are. Treat the student as an individual. Act as a resource for parents who want to do more for their child at home. Help the parents arrive at realistic educational goals for their child. Assist in developing worthwhile activities for work at home that will compliment the learning occurring in school. Provide reminders to parents about the student's strengths and successes at school. Present positive examples of the student's work.

Act as a resource when parents seek further information about epilepsy, organizations, services, etc. Encourage the parents' involvement with parent/advocacy groups. Be sure the parents know the school nurse and that they are knowledgeable about the school's emergency procedures. Obtain an update on the student's medications as well as drug changes, new side effects, etc. Discuss programs and strategies being used by educators with the child. Emphasize the school's self-esteem activities and the ways self-esteem enhancement could be carried through at home. Honor the confidentiality of the meeting.

And we must keep in mind the implications when Schneider (1988) stated that "Parents' worry, advice, and protection thus often magnified the significance of epilepsy and thus often magnified the significance of epilepsy in children's lives and could become a kind of control that isolated, restricted, and further disabled the children" (p. 71). Along the same idea, Wallace (1984) proposed the thought that a change in parental attitude toward a child after a seizure "might alter behaviour and opportunities for learning" (p. 18) on the part of the child.

Worthwhile literature for parents with a child with a disorder or disability can be found in a number of sources. The following list may serve as a beginning to a resource listing for parents:

Ehly, S.W., Conley, J.C., & Rosenthal, D.M. (1985). *Working with parents of exceptional children.* Columbus, OH: Charles E. Merrill.

Fewell, R.R., & Vadasy, P.F. (Eds.). (1986). *Families of handicapped children.* Austin, TX: Pro-Ed.

Gartner, A., Lipsky, D.K., & Turnbull, A.P. (1990). *Supporting families with a child with a disability.* Baltimore, MD: Paul H. Brookes.

Lambie, R., & Daniels-Mohring, D. (1993). *Family systems within educational contexts: Understanding students with special needs.* Denver: Love.

Simons, R. (1987). *After the tears: Parents talk about raising a child with a disability.* San Diego, CA: Harcourt Brace Jovanavich.

Stewart, J. C. (1986). *Counseling parents of exceptional children.* Columbus, OH: Charles E. Merrill.

Turnbull, H.R. & Turnbull, A.P. (1985). *Parents speak out: Then and now* (2nd ed.). Columbus, OH: Charles E. Merrill.

Turnbull, A.P. & Turnbull, H.R. (1990). *Families, professionals, and exceptionality: A special partnership* (2nd ed.). Columbus, OH: Charles E Merrill.

Magazine articles may also serve as useful resources for parents and families. For example, the pressures on the family and the challenges of parenting a child with epilepsy can be found in a number of articles, such as:

Goldman, J. (1985, July). Let's talk about seizures. Part I. Questions and answers for children. *Exceptional Parent,* 24–26, 28.

Hallsted, B.D. (1988, Nov./Dec.). Our son lives at home. *Exceptional Parent,* 18–24.

(No Author). (1979, Oct.). Mainstreaming and the child with epilepsy. *Exceptional Parent,* R9–R12.

Kelso, J. (1987, Nov./Dec.). Nurturing a special child. *Exceptional Parent,* 50–53.

RESOURCE:

The Exceptional Parent Magazine
120 State Street
Hackensack, NJ 07601-5421

Articles for parents and professionals on various aspects of caring for a child with disabilities and special health needs

FROM THE CLASSROOM:

[A school nurse states . . .] "Parents need to let the school staff know that a problem exists. They need to work with the nurse and any other staff member to keep the student in as normal a role as possible."

[A school nurse states . . .] "They [parents] thought that seizures meant she [student] was retarded."

RESOURCE:

Time Out For Families: Epilepsy And Respite Care
Epilepsy Foundation Of America

This booklet contains information about respite care for families; it discusses ways to obtain care and how the services should be evaluated; the booklet gives valuable tips, such as what do respite workers need from families; model respite care programs are presented.

RESOURCE:

Brothers and Sisters:
A Guide for Families of Children With Epilepsy
&
Issues and Answers: Exploring Your Possibilities—A Guide for Teens and Young People with Epilepsy
&
Issues and Answers—A Guide for Parents of Teens and Young Adults with Epilepsy

Contact:
Epilepsy Foundation of America
Phone: (800) EFA-1000

RESOURCE:

MUMS

150 Custer Court
Green Bay, Wisconsin

Mums is a national organization for parents or care providers of a child with a disability, disorder, chromosomal abnormality, or health condition. The organization provides support through a networking system that matches parents with other parents whose children have a similar condition. Parents can provide emotional support, medical information, and resources. A quarterly newsletter encourages parents to share information about current issues affecting the family.

There are no dues for parents, but a $15 fee is charged to professionals. Of particular interest is the fact that the group's data base consists of thousands of families dealing with over one thousand disorders and very rare syndromes.

RESOURCE:

Letter Exchange

Epilepsy U.S.A.
Epilepsy Foundation Of America
4351 Garden City Drive
Landover, MD 20785

Individuals have exchanged information and developed support systems through the published letters in the letter exchange in *Epilepsy U.S.A.* Students with epilepsy can develop pen pals and friends through the mail in the Junior Exchange of Letters. Letters from children must include a written and signed approval from the parent. The address above may also be used for the Junior Exchange.

FROM THE CLASSROOM:

[A school nurse states . . .] "I've found that parents of children with any disorder, not only seizures, are often well informed and often share information with me. In cases where parents need information, I share whatever resources I have with them."

Chapter 11

ADVOCACY AND CONCLUSION

SELF-ADVOCACY

Advocacy is the process of speaking and acting on behalf of a person with disabilities. It is a system that helps protect the rights and interests of an individual. In general, self-advocacy is interpreted to mean being able "to live as fully and independently as possible" (Brimer, 1990, p. 331).

Today, individuals with disabilities, including those with epilepsy, are speaking out and demanding their rights. They are openly stating their needs and protecting their own welfare and interests. "The central premise of self-advocacy is freedom to make choices" (Brimer, 1990, p. 343). Individuals with disabilities can and must act as their own advocates. "It [self-advocacy] is the parallel cry of self-determination by another group of disabled people rebelling against being long underestimated, deprived of choices, treated as eternal children, and thought to lead lesser lives" (Shapiro, 1993, p. 185).

STUDENT ADVOCACY

Student-to-student advocacy is a useful strategy for peers without disabilities to use for helping and guiding the interactions with other students with disabilities. Brimer (1990) noted that, while the original purpose was to increase interactions among students, student advocates can assume a variety of roles, such as assisting the student with a disability around the school, accompanying the student on field trips, or just being friends.

TEACHER ADVOCACY

The roles and responsibilities of teachers often require them to act as advocates (Brimer, 1990). In this capacity, teacher advocacy can be defined as speaking, working, and acting for a student in order to create positive change.

Educators should be knowledgeable about the many roles that can be played concerning advocacy and the change process. Ryndak (1994) provided a framework for roles that included change initiator, power sources, and change agents. "The change initiator is the individual who first identifies an unmet need and resolves to effect change until that need is met" (Ryndak, 1994, p. 253). This role could be played by a number of different individuals, including teachers, school administrators, family members and parent advocates. According to Ryndak (1994), "power sources are individuals with the capacity to effect change in either a positive or negative fashion" (p. 254). Potential power sources within and outside the school environment should be identified in relation to the type of change needed. "Change agents are individuals who actually conduct the activities through which the desired change will occur" (Ryndak, 1994, p. 255). Individuals, including teachers and other school personnel, can play this role in a manner to implement change.

A teacher in an advocate's role may take a position regarding a student's educational program or a student's right to participate in school activities. It may be the role of changing people's attitudes toward students with disabilities, or speaking out against barriers that limit students' full participation in school life. The teacher advocate may help create a school environment that is accepting of all students.

An educator can also provide the family with resources about epilepsy, as well as to direct the family to available local, state, and national services. The educator can act as a resource about epilepsy to other school personnel, such as cafeteria workers, administrators, school board members, custodians, bus drivers, etc.

The teacher can work with the family to develop their advocacy strategies, as well as to provide input into developing an appropriate school program for the student. A commitment to inclusion and mainstreaming, when appropriate, can be made for students with epilepsy.

Educators can provide relevant information about epilepsy to colleagues, especially concerning correct first-aid procedures for seizures. It is also important to communicate and maintain regular contact with the family, school nurse, and other medical personnel regarding the student's condition.

Educators must act as advocates since they are the ones who often are the first to identify students with epilepsy. They are the ones who spend six hours a day in close contact with the children. They are also the ones who can make a significant change in the school experience for students with epilepsy.

THE SILVER OWL AWARD

The Epilepsy Foundation of America honors educators who have observed the initial signs of seizures in a student, thus leading to the early identification of the disorder. According to the article "New E.F.A. Award" (1988), the Silver Owl Award will be given by Epilepsy Foundation affiliate offices, although the national office can also honor an educator. A primary purpose of the award is to bring attention to the importance of educators recognizing the early signs of seizure disorders.

FURTHER INFORMATION

Information on collaboration advocacy can be learned through a published series of manuals by the Epilepsy Foundation of America.

- *Partners in Advocacy: Understanding the Process*

  This booklet presents an overview of advocacy by the family and stresses the need for collaborating partnerships. The various types of advocacy are explained.

Partners in Advocacy: Family Action Guide

> This booklet gives families the information, skills, and strategies to become advocates. The specific steps in the advocacy process are described.

Partners in Advocacy: Affiliate Action Guide

> This booklet presents E.F.A. affiliates with strategies for advocacy.

Partners in Advocacy: Tools and Resources

> This booklet gives the reader resources (sample letters, publications, contacts, etc.) for advocacy. It includes a listing of state organizations concerned with individuals with disabilities.

One of the first resources to be recommended by the educator to the family would be the closest Epilepsy Foundation affiliate. The staff act as

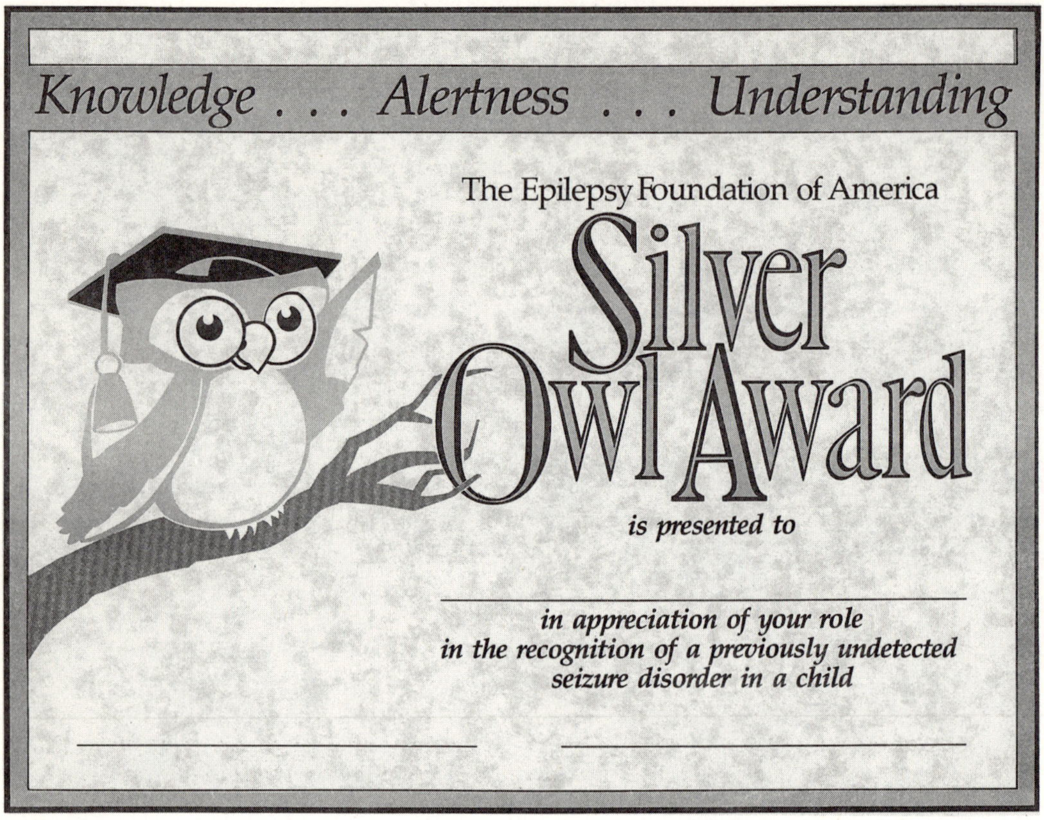
Knowledge . . . Alertness . . . Understanding
The Epilepsy Foundation of America
Silver Owl Award
is presented to
in appreciation of your role
in the recognition of a previously undetected
seizure disorder in a child

Figure 5. The Silver Owl Award. SOURCE: Epilepsy Foundation of America, Landover, Maryland.

local contacts who provide information, support, and resources to the family.

FROM THE CLASSROOM:

[A school nurse states . . .] "I think in general the public is more aware of, and sympathetic to, seizure disorders than twenty years ago. However, we need to work at dispelling fear: fear of having to deal with a seizure, and fear of the person who has seizures."

[A school nurse states . . .] "I see ignorance as an issue: on the part of parents telling their child not to tell anyone that they have a problem; on the part of staff, when a student seizes they

panic and force the student out of the room; and on the part of the student, who feels embarrassed and doesn't let anyone know that they have a problem."

"The parent teacher organization should also be inserviced and made aware that there are students with a seizure disorder and that the staff is able to deal with the problem. Reassurance is most important!"

"More publicity is needed! Let's get the problem out in the open! Bring it out of the closet!"

RESOURCE:

Numbers of useful videos are available. For example, there are videos for sale from the Epilepsy Foundation of America, with some available in Spanish.

"I Have Epilepsy Too!"
"Understanding Seizure Disorders"
"Understanding Complex Partial Seizures"
"Epilepsy and the Family"
"How Medicines Work"
"Epilepsy and the Teen Years"
"Living with Epilepsy"
"Take Another Look" (police video)
"Seizure Disorders and the School I"
"Seizure Disorders and the School II"
"School Planning for Children With Seizure Disorders"
"Seizure First Aid"
"And Life Goes On"
"The Rest of the Family"
"Meeting the Challenge"
"Voices from the Workplace"
"Driving and Epilepsy"

Contact the E.F.A. catalog and sales department for the most recent listing of videos.

E.F.A. Sales
4351 Garden City Drive
Landover, MD 20785

Credit Card Orders: (301) 577-0100
(800) 332-2070 (TDD)
FAX: (301) 577-9056

RESOURCE:

National Epilepsy Library

A free service for professionals; A comprehensive information base about epilepsy, including journal articles, books, papers, newsletters, reprints, and custom searches.
Phone: (800) EFA-4050

CONCLUSION

Advocacy for this population of students is an initial step for educators. Having relied on others in the past, educators now realize the importance of this role within their duties in schools. Recognizing the various needs of this population of students, educators are responding with appropriate actions.

There are large numbers of different types of disabilities, ranging in impact on the individual from mild to severe. Some disabilities are permanent and others are overcome. Some disabilities are hidden and some are episodic. Epilepsy is in this category, as it is not visible unless one is actually having a seizure, and it is a condition that appears at different times. It is this unpredictability of the condition that is one of the major concerns of educators. While life events in general have a degree of being unpredictable, it is truly emphasized in epilepsy.

The condition of epilepsy needs to be demystified within our schools. Knowledge, attitudes, and appropriate skills about the disorder are needed within the educational community. School personnel must become knowledgeable about this disorder as well as the needs of this population of students. It was with this concern that the book was written.

REFERENCES

Aldenkamp, A.P. (1994). Cognitive performance in learning disabled children with or without epilepsy. *Seizure, 3,* 13–21.

Aldenkamp, A.P., Alpherts, C.J., Dekker, M.J.H., & Overweg, J. (1990). Neuropsychological aspects of learning disabilities in epilepsy. *Epilepsia, 31,* 59–520.

American Academy of Pediatrics. (1983). Sports and the child with epilepsy. *Pediatrics, 72*(6), 884–885.

American Federation of Teachers. (1992). *The medically fragile child in the school setting.* Washington, DC: Author.

Americans with Disabilities Act of 1990: What should you know? (1990). *Exceptional Children, 57* (suppl.).

Annegers, J.F., Elvelback, L.R., Hauser, W.A., & Kuland, L.T. (1979). The risk of epilepsy following febrile convulsions. *Neurology, 24,* 297–303.

Anspaugh, D.J., Gilliland, M., & Anspaugh, S.J. (1980). The student with epilepsy. *Today's Education, 69,* 34GE-39GE.

Austin, J.K., & Fraser, R.T. (1993). Children with epilepsy: Their families and later vocational adjustments. *Issues in Epilepsy and Quality of Life,* 2–8.

Austin, J.K., Risinger, M.V., & Beckett, L.A. (1992). Correlates of behavior problems in children with epilepsy. *Epilepsia, 33*(6), 1115–1122.

Austin, J.K., Smith, M.S., Risinger, M.W., & McNelis, A.M. (1994). Childhood epilepsy and asthma: Comparison of quality of life. *Epilepsia, 35*(3), 608–615.

Baroff, G.S. (1991). *Developmental disabilities.* Austin, TX: Pro-Ed.

Batshaw, M.L., & Perrett, Y.M. (1986). *Children with handicaps.* Baltimore: Paul Brooks.

Baumer, J.H., David, T.J., Valentine, S.J., Roberts, J.E., & Hughes, B.R. (1981). Many parents think their child is dying when they have their first febrile convulsion. *Developmental Medicine and Child Neurology, 23,* 462–464.

Binnie, C.D., Channon, S., & Marston, D. (1990). Learning disabilities in epilepsy: Neurophysiological aspects. *Epilepsia, 31*(4), 52–58.

Birch, D. (1993, March 30). Hopkins reaps some remarkable results by using fatty foods to prevent seizures. *The Sun,* pp. 1, 8.

Beirne-Smith, M., Patton, J.R., & Ittenbach, R. (1994). *Mental retardation* (4th ed.). New York: Macmillan.

Bergen, D. (1991). The school child with epilepsy: How do we respond? *PTA Today, 16,* 18.

Best, S., Bigge, J., & Sirvis, B. (1990). Physical and health impairments. In N.G.

Harding and L. McCormick (Eds.), *Exceptional children and youth: An introduction to special education* (5th ed.) (pp. 283–284). Columbus, OH: Merrill.

Brimer, R.W. (1990). *Students with severe disabilities.* Mountain View, CA: Mayfield.

Buchanan, N., & Scambler, G. (1993). Epilepsy as an educational model. *Seizure, 2,* 45–48.

California State Council on Developmental Disabilities. (1992, August). *California epilepsy/seizure disorder needs assessment report.* Sacramento, CA: Author.

Camfield, R.P., Camfield, C.S., Shapiro, S.H., & Cummings, S.C. (1980). The first febrile seizure: Antipyretic instruction plus either phenobarbital or placebo to placebo to prevent recurrence. *Journal of Pediatrics, 97,* 16–21.

Camfield, C.S., Chaplin, S., Doyle, A.B., Shapiro, S.H., Cummings, C., & Camfield, P.R. (1979): Side effects of phenobarbital in toddlers: Behavioral and cognitive aspects. *Journal of Pediatrics, 95,* 361–365.

Carter, C.H. (1975). *Handbook of mental retardation syndromes* (3rd ed.). Springfield, IL: Charles C Thomas.

Cartwright, G.P., Cartwright, C.A., & Ward, M.E. (1984). *Educating special learners* (2nd ed.). Belmont, CA: Wadsworth.

Cavazzuti, G.B., Ferrari, P., & Lalla, M. (1984). Follow up study of 482 cases with convulsive disorder in the first year. *Developmental medicine and child neurology, 26,* 425–437.

Chavez, J.M., Guzman, B.L., Lee, H., & Mitchell, W.G. (1991). Academic underachievement in children with epilepsy. *Journal of Child Neurology, 6,* 65–72.

Consensus Statement. (1980). Febrile seizures: Long term management of children with fever associated seizures. *Pediatrics, 66,* 1009–1012.

Coulter, D. (1993). Epilepsy and mental retardation: An overview. *American Journal on Mental Retardation, 98,* 1–11.

Coulter, D.L., & Cerreto, M.C. (1993). *Enhancing the quality of life for the child with epilepsy and other disabilities.* Landover, MD: Epilepsy Foundation of America.

Cullum, C.M., Kuck, J., & Ruff, R.M. (1990). Neuropsychological assessment of traumatic brain injury in adults. In E.D. Bigler (Ed.), *Traumatic brain injury: Mechanisms of damage, assessment, intervention, and outcome* (pp. 129–163). Austin, TX: Pro-Ed.

Dam, M. (1990). Children with epilepsy: The effects of seizures, syndromes and etiological factors on cognitive functioning. *Epilepsia, 31*(suppl. 4), 526–529.

Devinsky, O. (1994). *A guide to understanding and living with epilepsy.* Philadelphia: F.A. Davis.

Diaz, A.S., Alegria, F.A., & Ferrando, L. (1986). Epilepticos en el colegio. *Archivos de nuerobiologia, 49,* 113–119.

Dilorio, C., Faherty, B., & Manteuffel, B. (1993). Learning needs of persons with epilepsy: A comparison of perceptions of persons with epilepsy, nurses and physicians. *Journal of Neuroscience Nursing, 25*(1), 22–29.

Disability Advisory Council of Australia. (1991–1992). The language of disability: Problems of politics and practice. *National Student Speech Language Hearing Association Journal, 19,* 55–60.

Dodrill, C.B. (1986). Correlates of generalized tonic-clonic seizures with intellectual, neuropsychological, emotional, and social functions in patients with epilepsy. *Epilepsia, 27*(4), 339–411.

Dodrill, C.B. (1982). Psychological assessment in epilepsy. In H. Sands (Ed.), *Epilepsy: A handbook for the mental health professional* (pp. 111–132). New York: Brunner and Mazel, Inc.

Dodson, E.W., Leppik, E., & Pedley, T.A. (1991). Are you up to date on seizures? *Patient Care, 25*(11), 162–166.

Dreifuss, F.E. (1988). What is epilepsy? In H. Reisner (Ed.), *Children with epilepsy* (pp. 1–32). Rockville, MD: Woodbine House.

Dreisbach, M., Ballard, M., Russo, D.C., & Schain, R.J. (1982). Educational intention for children with epilepsy. *Journal of Special Education, 16,* 111–121.

Driver law changes are less restrictive. (1994, August/September). *Epilepsy USA,* p. 9.

Driving & Epilepsy. (1993, January). *Epilepsy USA,* pp. 6–7.

Drotar, D., Baskiewicz, A., Irvin, N., Kennell, J.H., & Klaus, M.H. (1975). The adaptation of parents to the birth of an infant with a congenital malformation: A hypothetical model. *Pediatrics, 56,* 710–717.

Duchowny, M.S. (1987). Complex partial seizures of infancy. *Arch Neural, 44,* 911–914.

Duncan, J.S., Shorvon, S.D., & Trimble, M.R. (1990). Effects of removal of phenytoin, carabamazepine, and valproate of cognitive function. *Epilepsia, 31,* 584–591.

Edney, A.T.B. (1993). Dogs and human epilepsy. *The Veterinary Record,* 337–338.

Epilepsy Foundation of America. (1962). *Epilepsy: A survey of state laws.* Washington: Author.

Epilepsy Foundation of America. (1981). *The child with epilepsy at camp: A guide for counselors.* Landover, MD: Author.

Epilepsy Foundation of America. (1983). *Teaching students about epilepsy.* Landover, MD: Author.

Epilepsy Foundation of America. (1987). *Children and epilepsy: The teacher's role.* Landover, MD: Author.

Epilepsy Foundation of America. (1989). *Questions and answers about epilepsy.* Landover, MD: Author.

Epilepsy Foundation of America. (1991). *Issues and answers: A guide for parents of teens and young adults with epilepsy.* Landover, MD: Author.

Epilepsy Foundation of America. (1992a). *How to recognize and classify seizures and epilepsy* (2nd ed.). Landover, MD: Author.

Epilepsy Foundation of America. (1992b). *The legal rights of persons with epilepsy* (6th ed.). Landover, MD: Author.

Epilepsy Foundation of America. (1992c). *Seizure recognition and observation: A guide for allied health professionals.* Landover, MD: Author.

Erenberg, G. (1984). Febrile convulsions: A new look at our old problem. *Cleveland Clinic Quarterly, 51,* 279–282.

Ewing-Cobbs, L., & Fletcher, J.M. (1990). Neuropsychological assessment of traumatic brain injury in children. In E.D. Bigler (Ed.), *Traumatic brain injury* (pp. 107–128). Austin, TX: Pro-Ed.

Farwell, J.R., Dodrill, C.B., & Batzel, L.W. (1985). Neuropsychological abilities of children with epilepsy. *Epilepsia, 26*(5), 395–400.

Fishman, M.A. (1979). Febrile seizures: The treatment controversy. *The Journal of Pediatrics, 94,* 177–184.

Forness, S.R., and Kavale, K.A. (1988). Psychopharmacologic treatment: A note on classroom effects. *Journal of Learning Disabilities, 21,* 144–147.

Frank, B.B. (1985). Psychosocial aspects of educating epileptic children: Role for school psychologists. *School Psychology Review, 14*(2), 196–203.

Frank, J. (1990). Epilepsy: The school nurse's dilemma. *Journal of school health, 60*(1), 34–35.

Freeman, J.M., Vining, E.P.G., & Pillas, D. (1990). *Seizures and epilepsy in childhood: A guide for parents.* Baltimore, MD: Johns Hopkins.

Fuchs, D., & Fuchs, L.S. (1994). Inclusive schools movement and the radicalization of special education reform. *Exceptional Children, 60,* 294–309.

Gaddes, W.H. (1985). *Learning disabilities and brain function* (2nd ed.). New York: Springer-Verlag.

Gadow, K.D. (1979). *Children on medication: A primer for school personnel.* Reston, VA: The Council for Exceptional Children.

Gadow, K.D. (1982). School involvement in the treatment of seizural disorders. *Epilepsia, 23,* 215–224.

Garbe, K.C. (1990). Watering the shrinking violets: Teaching shy students. *Journal of school health, 60*(10), 509–510.

Gargiulo, R.M. (1985). *Working with parents of exceptional children: A guide for professionals.* Boston: Houghton Mifflin.

Gates, J. (1991). Epilepsy and sports participation. *The Physician and Sports Medicine, 19*(3), 99–104.

Gearheart, B., Mullem, C.R., & Gearheart, C. (1993). *Exceptional individuals: An introduction.* Belmont, CA: Cole Publishing.

Geist, H. (1962). *The etiology of idiopathic epilepsy.* New York: Exposition Press.

Giles, G.M., & Clark, W. (1993). *Brain injury rehabilitation: A neurofunctional approach.* San Diego, CA: Singular Publishing Group.

Gillberg, C. (1991). The treatment of epilepsy in autism. *Journal of Autism and Developmental Disorders, 21,* 61–77.

Goldberg, J.R. (1991). *What you can do about epilepsy.* New York: Dell Publishing.

Gorman, R.J., & Snead, O.C. (1979). Febrile seizures. *American Family Physician, 19,* 101–104.

Graf, W.D., Glass, S.T., Krauss, T.H., and Chatraian, G.E. (1992). Reflex seizures induced by playing video games: A clinical review and analysis of 26 patients with video games epilepsy. *Epilepsia, 33*(3), 126.

Grossman, R. (Ed.). (1983). *Manual on terminology and classification in mental retardation.* Washington DC: American Association on Mental Deficiency.

Guynn, J. (1983). The buddy system. *Journal of School Health, 53,* 624–625.

Hallahan, D.P., & Kauffman, J.M. (1991). *Exceptional children: Introduction to special education* (5th ed.). Englewood Cliffs, NJ: Prentice-Hall.

Hallahan, D.P., & Kauffman, J.M. (1994). *Exceptional children: Introduction to special education* (6th ed.). Needham Heights, MA: Allyn and Bacon.

Hammond, E.J., Uthman, B.M., Reid, S.A., & Wilder, B.J. (1992). Electrophysiological studies of cervical vagus nerve stimulation in humans I. EEG effects. *Epilepsia, 33*(6), 1013–1020.

Hansotia, P., & Broste, S.K. (1993). Epilepsy and traffic safety. *Epilepsia, 34*(5), 852–858.

Hardman, M.L., Drew, C.J., Egan, M.W., and Wolf, B. (1993). *Human exceptionality: Society, school, and family.* Boston: Allyn and Bacon.

Hartlage, L.C., & Green, J.B. (1972). The relation of parental attitudes to academic and social achievement in epileptic children. *Epilepsia, 13,* 21.

Hartshorne, T.S., & Boomer, L.W. (1993). Privacy of school records; What every special education teacher should know. *Teaching Exceptional Children, 25,* 32–35.

Hartshorne, J.C., & Byers, V.L. (1992). Impact of epilepsy on quality of life. *Journal of Neuroscience in Nursing, 24,* 24–29.

Hauser, W.A. (1994). The prevalence and incidence of convulsive disorder in children. *Epilepsia, 35*(suppl. 2), 51–56.

Hauser, W.A., & Hesdorffer, D.C. (1990). *Epilepsy: Frequency, causes, and consequences.* New York: Demos Publications.

Hayes, D.M., & Fors, S.W. (1990). Self esteem and health instruction: Challenges for curriculum development. *Journal of School Health, 60*(5), 208–211.

Hazelnis, A.E. (1991). *A study to identify and evaluate the concerns and issues facing public school nurses regarding children with seizures in Sullivan, Orange and Ulster Counties of New York State.* Unpublished Masters Project. New Paltz, NY: State University of New York.

Henriksen, O. (1990). Education and epilepsy: Assessment and remediation. *Epilepsia, 31*(suppl. 4), 521–525.

Hoar, P. (1984). The development of psychiatric disorder among school children with epilepsy. *Developmental Medicine and Child Neurology, 26,* 3–13.

Holder, L.K., Wernicke, J.F., & Tarver, B. (1992). Treatment of refractory partial seizures: Preliminary results of a controlled study. *Pacing and Clinical Electrophysiology, 15*(10), 1557–1571.

Hopkins, A. (1981). *Epilepsy—the facts.* New York: Oxford University Press.

Huberty, T.J., Austin, J.K., Risinger, M.W., & McNelis, A.M. (1992a). Classroom performance and adaptive skills in children with epilepsy. *Journal of School Psychology, 30,* 331–342.

Huberty, T.J., Austin, J.K., Risinger, M.W., & McNelis, A.M. (1992b). Relationship of selected seizure variables in children with epilepsy to performance on school administered tests. *Journal of Epilepsy, 5*(1), 10–16.

Hutt, S.J., Jackson, P., Belsham, H., and Higgins, J. (1968). Perceptual motor behavior in relation to blood phenobarbitone levels. A preliminary report. *Developmental Medicine and Child Neurology, 10,* 626–632.

Jambaque, I., Dellatolas, G., Dulac, O., & Signoret, J.L. (1992). Selective memory defects in children with partial epilepsy. *Epilepsia, 33,* 8.

Jan, J.E., Ziegler, R.G., & Erba, G. (1983). *Does your child have epilepsy?* Baltimore: University Park Press.

Jenkins, L.K. & Brown, S.W. (1992). Some issues in the assessment of epilepsy occuring in the context of learning disability in adults. *Seizure, 59*(1), 49–56.

Joachim, G. (1989). The school nurse as case manager for chronically ill children. *Journal of School Health, 59,* 406–407.

Kemp, A.M., & Sibert, J.R. (1993). Epilepsy in children and the risk of drowning. *Archives of Disease in Childhood, 68,* 684–685.

Kinnunen, E., & Wikstrom, J. (1986). Prevalence and prognosis of epilepsy in patients with multiple sclerosis. *Epilepsia, 27*(6), 729–733.

Kinsmen, S.L., Vining, E.P.G., Quaskey, S.H., Mellits, D., & Freeman, J.M. (1992). Efficacy of the ketogenic diet intractable seizure disorder: Review of 58 cases. *Epilepsia, 33*(6), 1132–1136.

Krier, J. (1993). Involvement of educational staff in the health care of medically fragile children. *Pediatric Nursing, 19*(3), 251–254.

Kroth, R. (1973). Behavioral Q sort as a diagnostic tool. *Academic Therapy, 8,* 317–330.

Lane, H. (1976). *The wild boy of Aveyron.* Cambridge: Harvard University Press.

Lebrun, Y. (1994). Ictal verbal behavior: A review. *Seizure, 3,* 45–54.

Leppik, I.E. (1990). Status epilepticus: The next decade. *Neurology, 40*(suppl. 12), 4–9.

Lesser, R.P., Lauders, H., Wyllie, E., Dinner, D.S., & Morris, H.H.III. (1986). Mental deterioration in epilepsy. *Epilepsia, 27(suppl. 2),* 5105–5123.

Litzinger, M.J., Duvall, B., & Little, P. (1993). Movement of individuals with complex epilepsy from an institution into the community: Seizure control and functional outcomes. *American Journal of Mental Retardation, 98,* 52–57.

Loiseau, P., Strube, E., & Broustet, D. (1983). Learning impairment in epileptic patients. *Epilepsia, 24,* 183–192.

Loring, D.W., & Meador, K.J. (1993). Cognitive and behavioral effects of antiepileptic drugs. *Issues in Epilepsy and Quality of Life,* 2–8.

Lynch, E.W., Lewis, R.B., & Murphy, D.S. (1992). Educational services for children with chronic illnesses: Perspectives of educators and families. *Exceptional Children, 59*(3), 210–220.

Marcus, J.C. (1993). Control of epilepsy in a mentally retarded population: Lack of correlation with IQ, neurological status, and electroencephalogram. *American Journal on Mental Retardation, 98,* 47–51.

McGowan, T. (1989). *Epilepsy.* New York: Franklin Watts.

Metrick, M.E., Ritter, F.J., Gates, J.R., Jacobs, M.P., Skare, S.S., & Loewenson, R.B. (1991). Nonepileptic events in childhood. *Epilepsia, 32*(3), 322–328.

Michael, R.J. (1992). Seizures: Teacher observations and record keeping. *Intervention in School and Clinic, 27*(4), 211–214.

Mitchell, M.E. (1992). Themes of concern for parents of children with epilepsy. *Epilepsia, 33*(suppl. 3), 15.

Mitchell, W.G., Chavez, J.M., Lee, H., & Guzman, B.L. (1991). Academic underachievement in children with epilepsy. *Journal of Child Neurology, 6*(1), 65–72.

Murphy, J.V., & Dekharghani, F. (1994). Diagnosis of childhood seizure disorder. *Epilepsia, 35*(2), 57–517.

National Information Center for Children and Youth with Disabilities. (1991). *Related services for school-aged children with disabilities.* Washington, DC: Author.

New E.F.A. award to honor teachers. (1988, May–June). *National Spokesman,* p. 3.

Neurologic Disorders. (1984). Springhouse, PA: Springhouse.

Obrzut, J.E., & Hynd, G.W. (1987). Cognitive dysfunction and psychoeducational assessment in traumatic brain injury. In E.D. Bigler (Ed.), *Traumatic brain injury: Mechanisms of damage, assessment, intervention, and outcome* (pp. 165–180). Austin, TX: Pro-Ed.

O'Leary, D.S., Lovell, M.R., & Sackelares, J.C. (1983). Effects of age of onset of partial and generalized seizures on neuropsychological performance in children. *Journal of Nervous and Mental Disease, 171*(10), 624–629.

Oliver, J. (Ed.). (1983). *Teaching students about epilepsy.* Portland, OR: Good Samaritan Hospital and Medical Center.

Olson, I., & Campenhausen, G. (1993). Sound adjustment in young adults with absence seizures. *Epilepsia, 34*(5), 846–851.

Osborne, A.G., & Dimattia, P. (1994). The IDEA's least restrictive environment mandate: Legal implications. *Exceptional Children, 61*(1), 6–14.

Ozuna, J. (1993). Ethical dilemmas in epilepsy and driving. *Journal of Epilepsy, 6,* 185–188.

Pary, R. (1993). Mental retardation, mental illness, and seizure diagnosis. *American Journal of Mental Retardation, 98,* 58–62.

Patton, J.R., Payne, J.S., & Beirne-Smith, M. (1990). *Mental retardation.* New York: Merrill.

Perske, R. (1972). *The dignity of risk.* Toronto: National Institute of Mental Retardation.

Poindexter, A.R., Berglund, J.A., & Kolstoe, P.D. (1993). Changes in antiepileptic drug prescribing patterns in large institutions: Preliminary results of a five year experience. *American Journal on Mental Retardation, 98,* 34–40.

Pope, W.A., McHale, S.M., & Craighead, W.E. (1988). *Self esteem enhancement with children and adolescents.* New York: Pergamon Press.

Porter, R.J. (1993). The absence epilepsies. *Epilepsia, 34*(Suppl. 3), 542–548.

Potolicchio, S. (1992, Feb.). Understanding epilepsy. *N.E.A. Today,* 13.

Pressey, S.L., & Pressey, L.C. (1927). *Mental abnormality and deficiency.* New York: Macmillan.

Reid, R., Maag, J.W., & Vasa, S.F. (1993). Attention deficit hyperactivity disorder, a disability category: A critique. *Exceptional Children, 60,* 198–214.

Related Services for School Aged Children with Disabilities (vol. 1). (1991). National Information Center for Children and Youth with Disabilities. Washington, DC.

Reynolds, C.R., & Mann, L. (1987). *Encyclopedia of special education* (Vol. 2). New York: John Wiley and Sons.

Ridgeway, G., & Like, M. (1991). Demystifying tonic-clonic seizures. *Nursing 91, 21*(11), 62–64.

Rodin, E.A., Schmaltz, S., & Twitty, G. (1986). Intellectual functions of patients with childhood onset epilepsy. *Developmental Medicine and Neurology, 28,* 25–33.

Rogers, J. (1993, May). The inclusion revolution. *Research bulletin.* Phi Delta Kappa center for evaluation, development, and research.

Rowland, T.W. (1990). *Exercise and children's health.* Champaign, IL: Human Kinetics Books.

Ryndak, D.L. (1994). *A systems change approach to advocacy.* Boston: Allyn and Bacon.

Salend, S.J. (1994). *Effective mainstreaming: Creating inclusive classrooms* (2nd ed.). New York: Macmillan.

Salinsky, M.C., and Burcheil, K.J. (1993). Vagus nerve stimulation has no effect on awake eeg rhythms in humans. *Epilepsia, 34*(2), 299–304.

Sands, H. (1982). *Epilepsy: A handbook for the mental health professional.* New York: Brunner/Mazel.

Sands, H., & Minters, F.C. (1977). *The epilepsy factbook.* New York: Charles Silvers Books.

Santilli, N., Dodson, W.E., and Walton, A.V. (1991). *Students with seizures: A manual for school nurses.* Cedar Grove, NJ: Health Scan.

Savage, R.C. (1988). Introduction to educational issues for students who have suffered traumatic brain injury. In R.C. Savage & G.F. Wolcott (Eds.), *An educator's manual: What educator's need to know about students with traumatic brain injury* (pp. 1–9). Southborough, MA: National Head Injury Foundation.

Schachter, S.C. (1995). *The brainstorms companion.* New York: Raven Press.

Schneider, J.W. (1988). Disability as a moral experience: Epilepsy and self in routine relationships. *Journal of Social Issues, 44,* 63–78.

Schwartz, R.H., Eaton, J., Bower, B.D., & Aynsley-Green, A. (1989). Ketogenic diets in the treatment of epilepsy: Short term clinical effects. *Developmental Medicine and Child Neurology, 31*(2), 145–151.

Schwartz, R.M., Boyes, S., & Aynsley-Green, H. (1989). Ketogenic diets in the treatment of epilepsy: Short term clinical effects. *Developmental Medicine and Child Neurology, 31*(2), 152–168.

Scott, D. (1969). *About epilepsy.* New York: International Universities Press.

Scheidmann, N.V. (1931). *The psychology of exceptional children* (vol. 1). New York: Houghton Mifflin.

Seidenberg, M., Beck, N., Geisser, M., Giordani, B., Sackellaress, J.C., Berent, S., Dreifuss, F.E., & Boll, T.J. (1986). Academic achievement of children with epilepsy. *Epilepsia, 27*(6), 753–759.

Seligman, M., & Datliong, R.B. (1989). *Ordinary families, special children.* New York: Guilford.

Sexton, S.B., & Madan-Swain, A. (1993). School reentry for the child with chronic illness. *Journal of Learning Disabilities, 26*(2), 115–125, 137.

Shapiro, J.P. (1993). *No pity.* New York: Times Books.

Shea, T.M., & Bauer, A.M. (1994). *Learners with disabilities.* Madison, WI: Brown and Benchmark.

Sillanpaa, M. (1992). Epilepsy in children: Prevalence, disability, and handicap. *Epilepsia, 33*(3), 444–449.

Silver Owls. (1990, May). *National Spokesman,* p. 4.

Singe, B.K., & Towle, P.O. (1993). Antiepileptic drug status in adult outpatients with mental retardation. *American Journal on Mental Retardation, 98,* 41–46.

Slapin, B., Lessing, J., & Belkind, E. (1987). *Books without bias: A guide to evaluating children's literature for handicapism.* Berkeley, CA: Kids Project.

Smith, C.R. (1991). *Learning disabilities* (2nd ed.). Boston: Allyn and Bacon.

Smith, D.D., & Luckasson, R. (1992). *Introduction to special education.* Needham Heights, MA: Allyn and Bacon.

Smith, J.A., & Wallace, S.J. (1982). Febrile convulsions: Intellectual progress in relation to anticonvulsant therapy and recurrence of fits. *Archives of Disease in Childhood, 57,* 104–107.

Snyder, M. (1993). Revised epilepsy stressor inventory. *Journal of Neuroscience in Nursing, 25,* 9–13.

Spitz, M.C. (1992). Severe burns as a consequence of seizures in patients with epilepsy. *Epilepsia, 33,* 103–107.

Stafstrom, C.E. (1993). Epilepsy in Down's syndrome: Clinical aspects and neurological considerations. *American Journal on Mental Retardation, 98,* 12–26.

Stedman, J., Van Heyningen, R., & Lindsay, J. (1982). Educational underachievement and epilepsy: A study of children from normal schools admitted to a special hospital for epilepsy. *Early Child Development and Care, 9,* 52–65.

Stem, B., & Test, D.W. (1989). Teaching first aid skills in the classroom. *Teaching Exceptional Children, 22,* 10–12.

Strixrud, W.R. (1988). Helping your child develop self esteem. In H. Reisner (Ed.), *Children with epilepsy* (pp. 83–112). Rockville, MD: Woodbine House.

Sullivan, R. (1994, January 12). Some seizures tied to flashing lights. *The New York Times,* p. c12.

Sunder, T.R., and Davis, R. (1992). Epileptic syndrome in a multihandicapped population. *Epilepsia, 33*(Suppl. 3), 69–70.

Svoboda, W.B. (1979). *Learning about epilepsy.* Baltimore: University Park Press.

Terry, R.S., Tarver, W.B., & Zabara, J. (1991). The implantable neurocybernetic prosthesis system. *Cyberonics, 14,* 86–93.

Tower, D.B. (1960). *Neurochemistry of epilepsy.* Springfield, IL: Charles C Thomas.

Treiman, D.M. (1986). Epilepsy and violence: Medical and legal issues. *Epilepsia, 27*(Suppl. 2), s77–s104.

Trimble, M.R. (1990). Antiepileptic drugs, cognitive function, and behavior in children: Evidence from recent studies. *Epilepsia, 31*(4), 530–534.

Trippi, J. (1989). Monitoring children on medication. *Transitions in Mental Retardation, 4,* 231–249.

United States Office of Education. (1977). Implementation of part B of the Education of the Handicapped Act. *Federal Register, 42,* 42474–42518.

U.S. Dept. of Health Education and Welfare. (1961). *The child with epilepsy.* Children's Bureau Folder, *35.*

Valente, W.D. (1980). *Law in the schools.* Columbus, OH: Charles E. Merrill.

Vining, E.P.G. (1987). Cognitive dysfunction associated with antiepileptic drug therapy. *Epilepsia, 28*(Suppl. 2), 518–522.

Vining, E.P.G., Mellits, E.D., & Dorsen, M.M. (1987). Psychological and behavioral effects of antiepileptic drugs in children: A double-blind comparison between phenobarbital and valproic acid. *Pediatrics, 80,* 165–174.

Vermeulen, J., Kortstee, S., Alpherts, W., & Aldenkamp, A. (1994). Cognitive performance in learning disabled children with and without epilepsy. *Seizure, 3*(1), 13–21.

Volkmar, F.R., & Nelson, D.S. (1990). Seizure disorders in autism. *Journal of the American Academy of Child and Adolescent Psychiatry, 29*(1), 127–129.

Wagman, R.J. (1983). *The medical and health encyclopedia.* Chicago: J.G. Ferguson.

Walker, J., & Rowan, J. (1993). Nonepileptic (pseudoepileptic) seizures (NES). *Issues in Epilepsy and Quality of Life,* 2–8.

Wallace, S. (1984). Febrile convulsions: Their significance for later intellectual development and behavior. *Journal of Child Psychology and Psychiatry, 25*(1), 15–21.

Wallace, S.J., & Cull, A.M. (1979). Long term psychological outlook for children whose first fit occurs with fever. *Developmental Medicine and Child Neurology, 21,* 28–40.

Wilder, B.J., Uthman, B.M., & Hammond, E.J. (1991). Vagal stimulation for control of complex partial seizures in medically refractory epileptic patients. *Cyberonics, 14,* 108–115.

Wolf, S., Forsythe, A., Stunden, A., Freidman, R., & Diamond, H. (1981). Long-term effect of phenobarbital on cognitive function in children with febrile convulsions. *Pediatrics, 68*(6), 820–823.

Wolfensberger, W. (1972). *The principal of normalization in human services.* Toronto: National Institute on Mental Retardation.

Wolfensberger, W. (1985). An overview of social role valorization and some reflections on elderly mentally retarded persons. In M.P. Janicki and H.M. Wisniewski (Eds.), *Aging and developmental disabilities: Issues and approaches* (pp. 61–76). Baltimore: Paul H. Brookes.

Wyllie, E. (Ed.). (1993). *The treatment of epilepsy: Principles and practice.* Philadelphia: Lea and Febiger.

Yard, G., & Thurman, R. (1982). Seizure disorders and emotionally disturbed children and youth: An inservice training model. *Behavior Disorders, 7*(2), 86–90.

Zeigler, R.G. (1983). The child with epilepsy: Psychotherapy and counseling. In H. Sands (Ed.), *Epilepsy* (pp. 158–188). New York: Brunner and Mazel.

AUTHOR INDEX

SUBJECT INDEX

Q

R

S

T

U

V